the creative will

*an exhibition of works
by thirty-one artists
with multiple sclerosis*

PROJECT REMBRANDT® X

NATIONAL MS SOCIETY

POMEGRANATE ARTBOOKS • SAN FRANCISCO

Dedicated to the memory of Lowell Nesbitt, 1933–1993.

Published by Pomegranate Artbooks
Box 6099, Rohnert Park, California 94927

© 1993 National Multiple Sclerosis Society

ISBN 1-56640-597-1
Library of Congress Catalog Card Number 93-84778

Designed by Bonnie Smetts Design

Printed in Korea

project rembrandt is the National MS Society's juried national biennial art exhibition program for professional artists who have multiple sclerosis—a chronic, often debilitating disease of the central nervous system that usually strikes in early adulthood and for which there is as yet no cure.

Thirty-one artists were chosen to participate in *The Creative Will*, the tenth anniversary exhibition of Project Rembrandt. From seventeen states extending from Oregon to Florida and New Mexico to New York, these artists have works in important private and public collections worldwide. They were selected from nearly two hundred entrants by a distinguished jury: Diane Waldman, deputy director and senior curator of the Solomon R. Guggenheim Museum; Paul J. Smith, director emeritus of the American Craft Museum and independent curator; and Lowell Nesbitt, renowned artist and cochairman of the Project Rembrandt national advisory committee.

After the finalists were selected, their biographical materials were reviewed, and it was revealed that the level of disability among them ran the gamut. One painter has such limited mobility that she paints with a brush in her mouth. Some use aids, such as wheelchairs, canes or electric carts. Still others suffer from serious vision problems and/or severe fatigue, but outwardly manifest few obvious signs of the disease. Each meets the challenges of multiple sclerosis on his or her own terms, adapting, persevering, accommodating and ultimately creating art out of life.

By providing a forum for the work of these artists the Society strives to build awareness about MS and its impact on people's lives, to foster public support for MS research and services, and to demonstrate that *disability is not synonymous with inability* (the Project Rembrandt credo). By consenting to show their work as a special group, the Project Rembrandt artists not only educate the public but help to encourage others with the disease, or other disabilities or obstacles, to pursue dreams of their own.

Dustin Hoffman, Carol Lawrence, Julie Andrews, Jean Kennedy-Smith, Anthony Quinn, Philip Pearlstein, John Chamberlain, Malcolm Morley and J. Carter Brown, among many others, support the program. It is the hope of the Society that you, too, will receive inspiration and enjoyment from the art of *The Creative Will* and want to become involved with the MS cause.

For further information about MS and the National MS Society, see page 96.

jurors' statement

The Creative Will: Project Rembrandt X is the most recent in a unique series of fine contemporary art exhibitions that both raise awareness about MS and celebrate artistic achievements.

The strength of the program arises from the strength of the art; the judging was in no way compromised by the special classification of the artists. Artists with MS were invited to submit slides of up to ten works in any visual fine art medium. Our mission as jury members was exacting: we were to choose the best works by the best artists in combination to create a balanced, interesting art exhibition, which both represented the scope of each artist's work and reflected the range of mediums submitted.

We are pleased to report that the quality of submissions within each discipline was high. This in conjunction with the fact that nearly half of the artists who entered did so for the first time—even though the program has been in existence for ten years—has led us to conclude that Project Rembrandt continues to grow and improve. We believe that the strict standards of the competition have been key in attracting outstanding talent over the years.

Although we had been requested to select only twenty artists, in the end we chose thirty-one, feeling that any additional cuts would be arbitrary. All are established professionals, and while some may not have achieved national prominence yet, their originality, technique and/or particular sensibility cause the viewer to take note. We look forward to observing their careers continue to develop.

We also congratulate all two hundred artists who entered The Creative Will competition for their ability to surmount the numerous and disparate challenges of MS. You are the heart of the program.

Lowell Nesbitt, *artist*
Paul J. Smith, *director emeritus, American Craft Museum, and independent curator*
Diane Waldman, *deputy director and senior curator, Solomon R. Guggenheim Museum*

artists

Bess C. Bonner
Karen L. De Witt
Laszlo Dus
Victoria (Tori) Ellison
Leah Finch
Phoebe Fuller-Graham
Judith J. Hahn
John M. Hall
Angelina M. A. Hekking
Thomas W. Hollender
Robert Otis Holter
Carol Hunt
James Iatridis
Dina Kawer
Frieda King
Rona Ginn Klein
Jessie Jane Lewis
Linda L. Longo-Muth
Marty Manning
Thomas Martin
Ruby McLain
Surel Mitchell
Debra Norby
Mary O'Hara Gregory
Jeana Sirabella
Karen G. Stone
Charles Strouchler
James Uhl
Lorna R. Warden
Kay Yasutome
Hugh C. Yorty

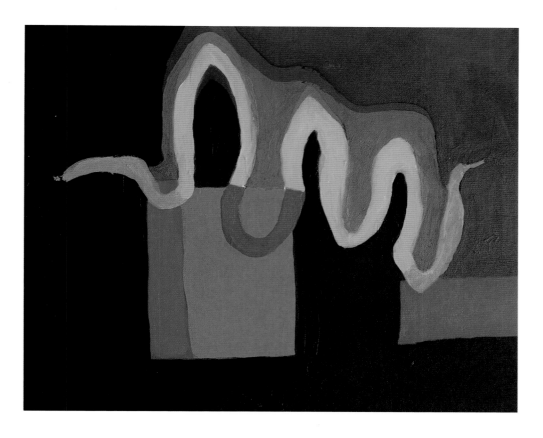

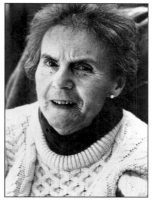

"If you find it necessary to express yourself with line, form and color, no matter what happens, you will find a way."

Bess C. Bonner

Colorado Springs, Colorado

MS cut short Bess Bonner's career as a medical illustrator at thirty-five. Eighteen years later she visited Mexico and was inspired to paint by "the lushness of the colors and the climate and the warmth of the people." Unable to use her hands, she taught herself to paint with a brush in her mouth. "One tends to think that artists use their hands to express themselves," she says, "but since creative ideas originate in the mind, it does not matter [how] the paint is applied." Bonner's abstract oil paintings result from recent experimentation. Her prize-winning work appears in juried and invitational exhibits nationwide.

Tahola, 1992. Oil on canvas, 16 x 20 in.

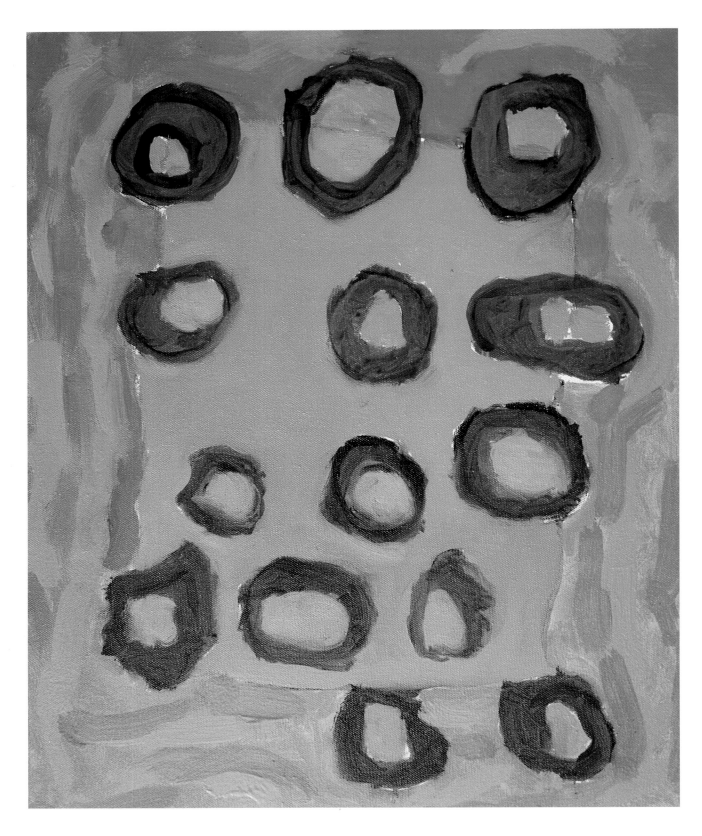

Kalama, 1992. Oil on canvas, 20 x 16 in.

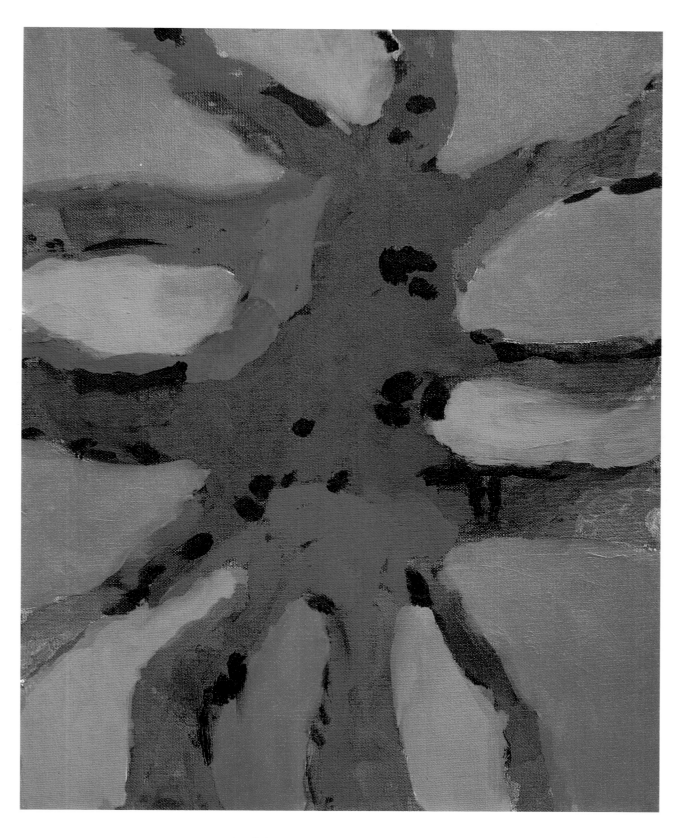

Unidentified Sea Creature, 1992. Oil on canvas, 20 x 16 in.

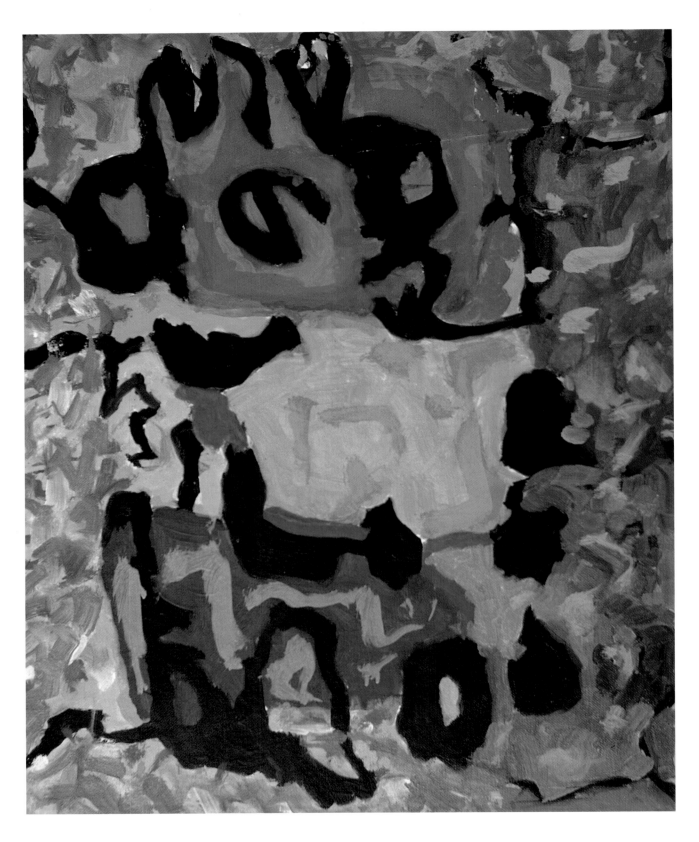

Spuzzum, 1992. Oil on canvas, 20 x 16 in.

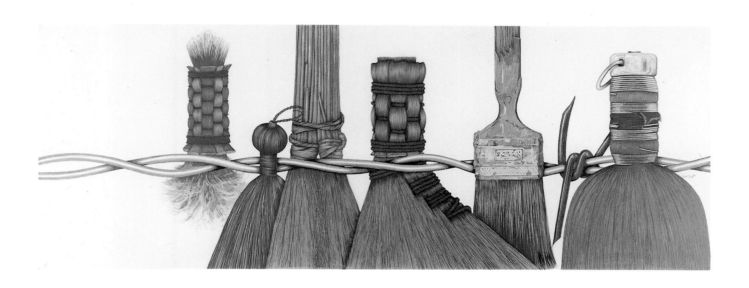

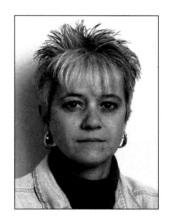

"I am not trying to 'tell a story' or 'set a mood,' but rather to expose an otherwise unseen, unnoticed facet of my subject."

Karen L. De Witt

Park Forest, Illinois

On receiving her M.F.A. degree from Southern Illinois University in 1977, Karen De Witt set a goal to become a full-time artist by age forty. She spent the next ten years positioning herself as a professional artist, meanwhile developing the framing business she cocreated, Frame Masters, Ltd. In 1987, De Witt was diagnosed with MS. Only three years away from her fortieth birthday, she felt she could no longer postpone her art career and has spent the last five years producing work, entering competitions and exhibiting. Today De Witt is represented by galleries in Chicago, Minneapolis and San Francisco. Her work is in major collections worldwide.

The Line Up, 1992. Graphite, pastel and prisma on paper, 21 x 46 in. Collection of Ann Benson.

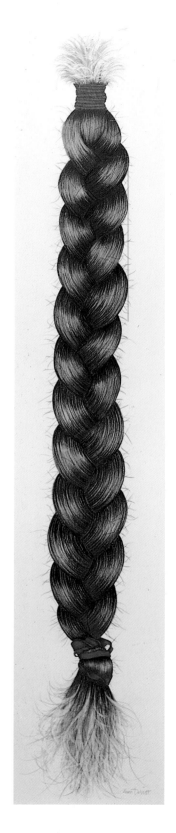

I feel so fine when they compare mine to Dine, 1992. Graphite, pastel and prisma on paper, 46 x 13½ in.

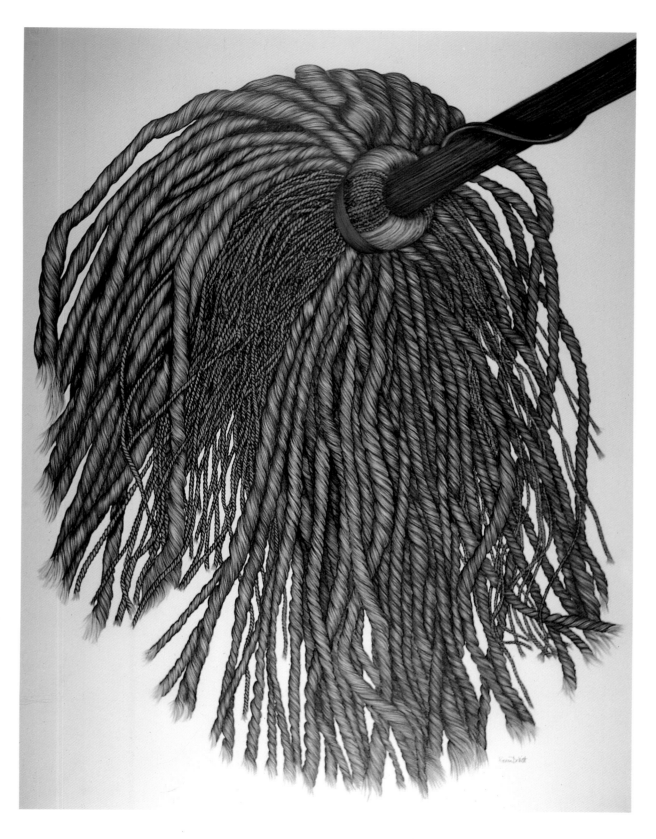

Mophead III, 1992. Graphite, pastel and prisma on paper, 46 x 36 in.

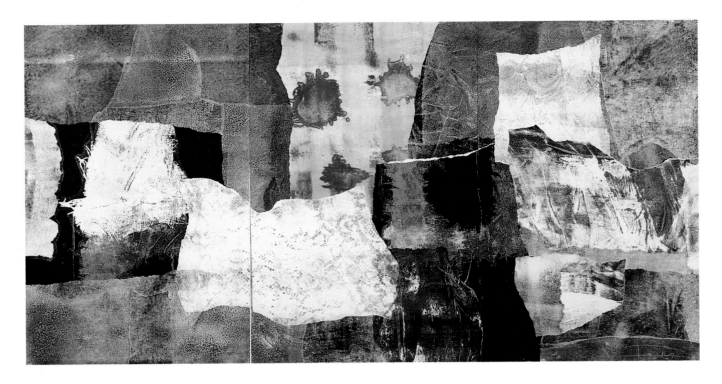

Laszlo Dus

Brecksville, Ohio

"I cannot talk about my art in a couple of sentences and I would not do it in more."

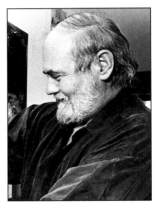

Laszlo Dus began his distinguished art career in Hungary, his native country. Singled out for his artistic aptitude as a boy, he was trained in national art schools in Budapest. After exhibiting widely throughout eastern and western Europe in the 1960s, Dus immigrated to the United States in 1974. His paintings, lithographs, monoprints, silkscreens and collages are found in the permanent collections of the Metropolitan Museum of Art, the National Gallery of Fine Arts and the Art Institute of Chicago, among other important institutions. He was diagnosed with MS in 1989.

Untitled (triptych), 1989. Acrylic on canvas, 36 x 69 in.

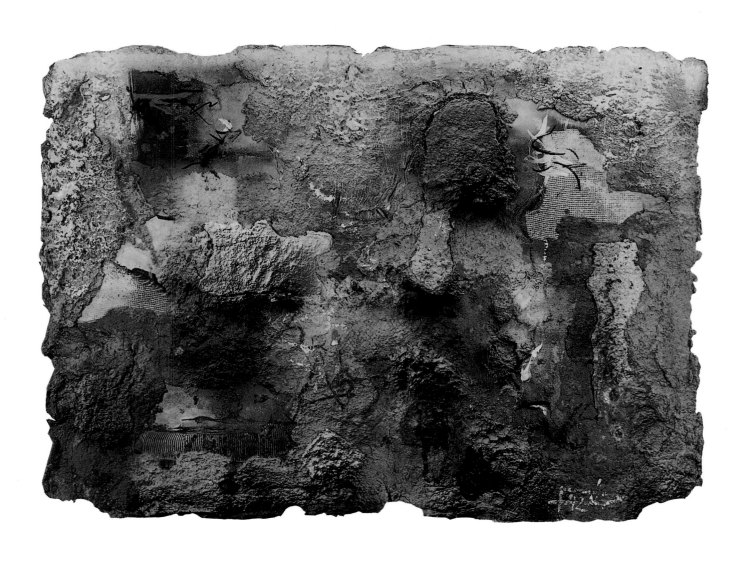

Untitled, 1989. Handmade paper, 27 x 37 in.

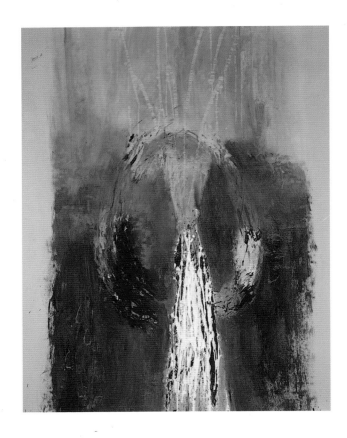

Victoria (Tori) Ellison

Brooklyn, New York

"My desire is to visualize processes of transformation, both physical and abstract, external and internal."

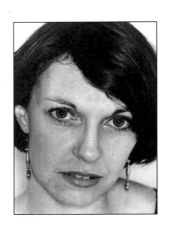

Tori Ellison—a painter, sculptor and installation artist—studied at Cranbrook Academy of Art and the School of Visual Arts, New York City, receiving her M.F.A. degree in 1987. She has been awarded fellowships from the MacDowell Colony and Blue Mountain Art Center as well as artist residencies at Artpark, Lewiston, New York, and in the New York City Public Schools, through Andy Warhol Foundation funding. Her work is exhibited bicoastally and appears in collections internationally. Ellison also teaches art to students in grade school through college and is an editor for the Solomon R. Guggenheim Museum and Rizzoli International Publications. She was diagnosed with MS in 1991.

Untitled, 1987. Acrylic on paper, 60 x 48 in.

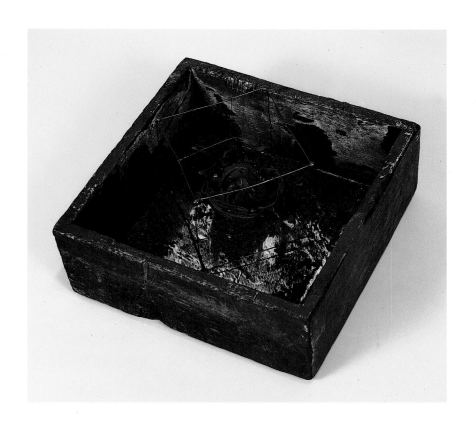

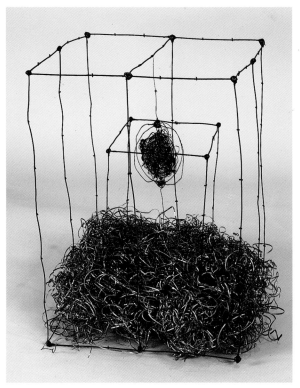

Untitled, 1991. Wood, mirror, ash, wire, paint and plastic tubing, 5 x 13 x 13 in. (top)
Untitled, 1991. Wire, paint and steel shavings, 18 x 12 x 12 in. (bottom)

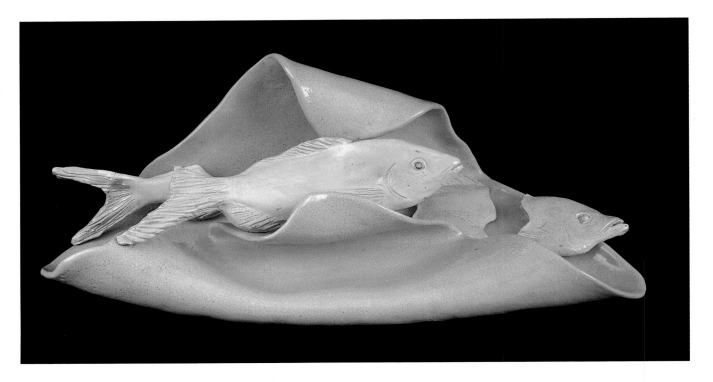

Leah Finch

Margate, Florida

"Just touching the clay body itself often inspires me to create; it is the medium that feels most natural to me."

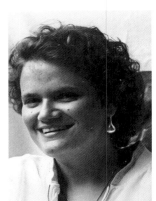

"Having multiple sclerosis can make a determined person very creative," says Leah Finch. She was diagnosed with MS at twenty-two and almost immediately had little control from the neck down. Unable to paint as she had been, she took a class in ceramic sculpture that focused on people with disabilities and has worked in that medium ever since. In spite of MS Finch went on to earn her B.F.A. degree from the University of San Francisco and the Academy of Art College, San Francisco, by taking one class at a time over eight years. She is now working toward a master's degree in speech and language pathology at Novo University, Miami.

Untitled, 1992. Low fire ceramics, 12 x 23 x 18 in.

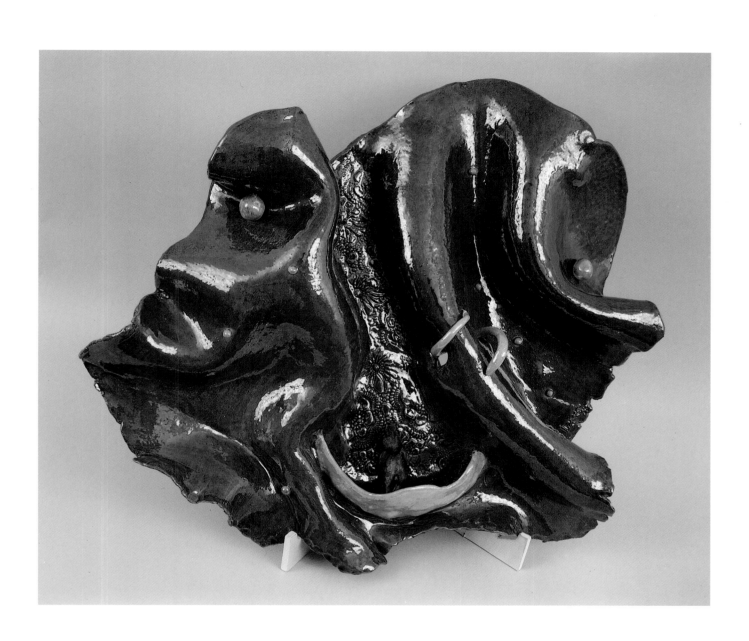

Cradle of Sustenance, 1992. Low fire ceramics, 16 x 18 x 4 in.

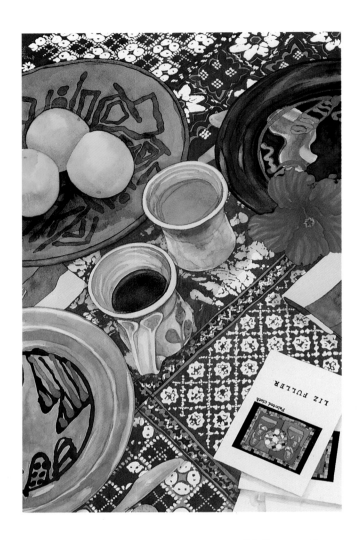

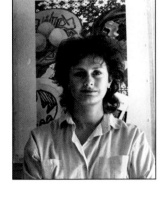

"It is the composition . . . that, for me, defines a successful work. . . . I like to activate chosen shapes and forms with color and designs."

Phoebe Fuller-Graham

Irvine, California

Art is part of Phoebe Fuller-Graham's heritage: both her parents are artists, as were several of her ancestors. In 1982 she received a B.A. degree in studio art from the University of California, Riverside. "Shape and form," she explains, ". . . color and surface design have always been my interest. . . . When I juxtapose and overlap surface patterns, form is further revealed by the edges and lines. And movement flows along these lines." Her works on paper are exhibited in galleries and businesses throughout California. She was diagnosed with MS at thirty-three in 1988.

Summer Still Life on Batik #1, 1992. Watercolor on paper, 23¾ x 15¼ in.

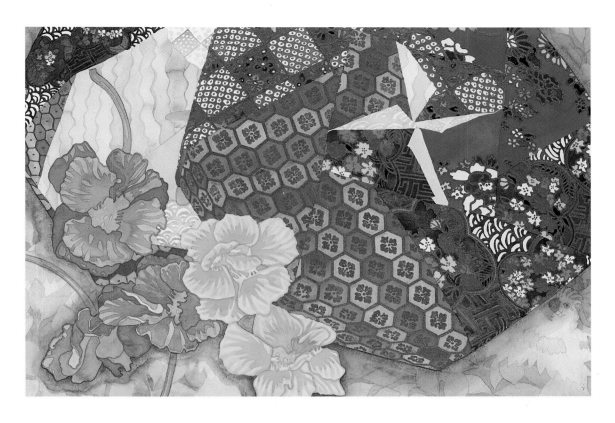

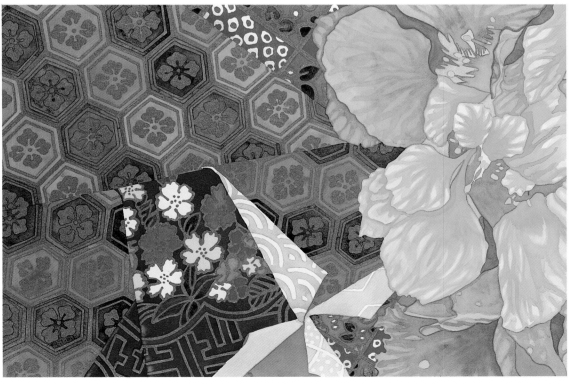

Origami Box #1, 1992. Watercolor on paper, 28¼ x 36 in. (top) *Origami Box #2,* 1992. Watercolor on paper, 28¼ x 36 in. (bottom)

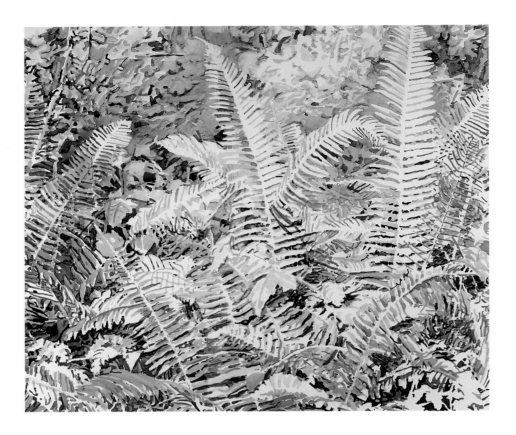

Judith J. Hahn

Woodinville, Washington

"My work now deals with the light on things in the woods, fields and waters of my beautiful Pacific Northwest home."

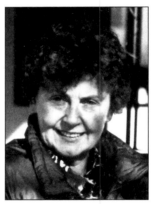

Judith Hahn has been a professional painter and print-maker for the past thirty years. She is proud that she has been able to meld a full-time art career, which has included teaching, with a full family and community life. Her increasing disability caused by chronic-progressive MS, diagnosed in 1980, has intensified her involvement with her art. Post-MS, her work has broadened from intaglio printing to a wide range of realistic paintings on canvas. Hahn's prints and paintings are found in major collections nationwide, including those of the Brooklyn Museum and the Smithsonian Institution, Washington, D.C.

Ferns I, 1992. Watercolor on paper, 27 x 33 in.

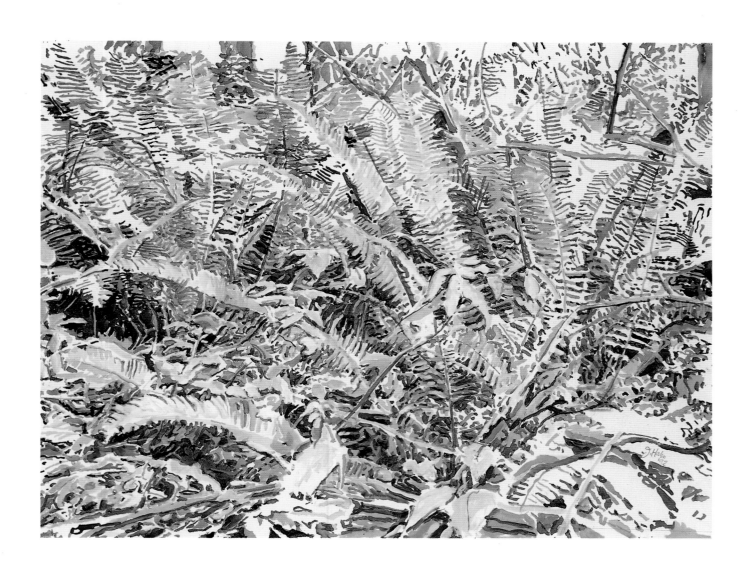

Ferns II, 1992. Watercolor on paper, 33 x 37 in.

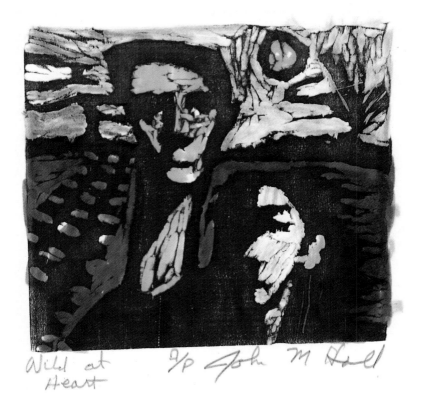

Wild at Heart 9/p John M Hall

John M. Hall

San Jose, California

"Creating a new piece of art takes the pain, fear and anxiety inside of me and turns it into hope, relief and 'Art for Life.'"

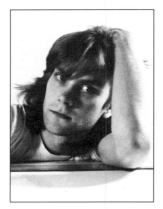

Soon after John Hall moved west from a small Illinois town, he established himself in the underground art communities of San Jose and Santa Cruz. A graphic artist for a northern California entertainment weekly, he produced and exhibited his work and published a magazine, *Telepathic Reader,* with several Bay Area artists. After developing MS in 1989, vision problems impaired his ability to keep his job, and he became a homemaker for his wife and children. He has since embraced new art forms through which he expresses himself: woodcuts and boldly colored paintings.

Wild At Heart, 1991. Watercolor woodcut, 6 x 6 in.

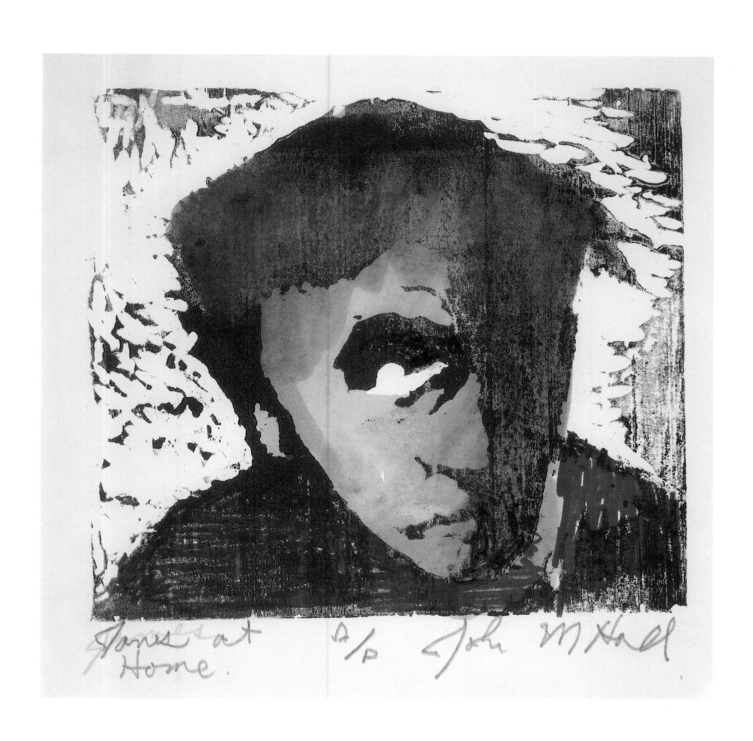

James At Home, 1991. Watercolor woodcut, 6 x 6 in.

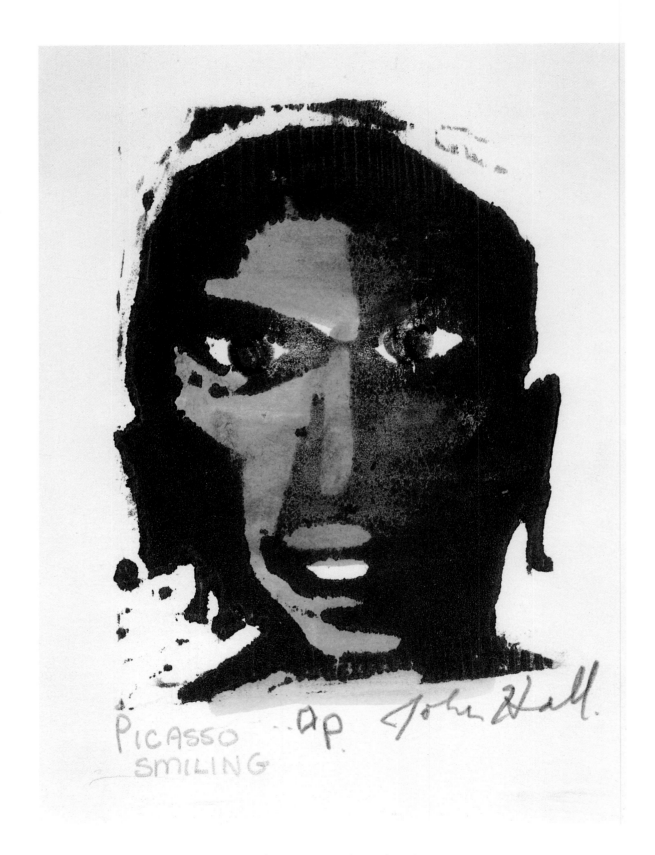

Picasso Smiling, 1991. Watercolor woodcut, 5½ x 4 in.

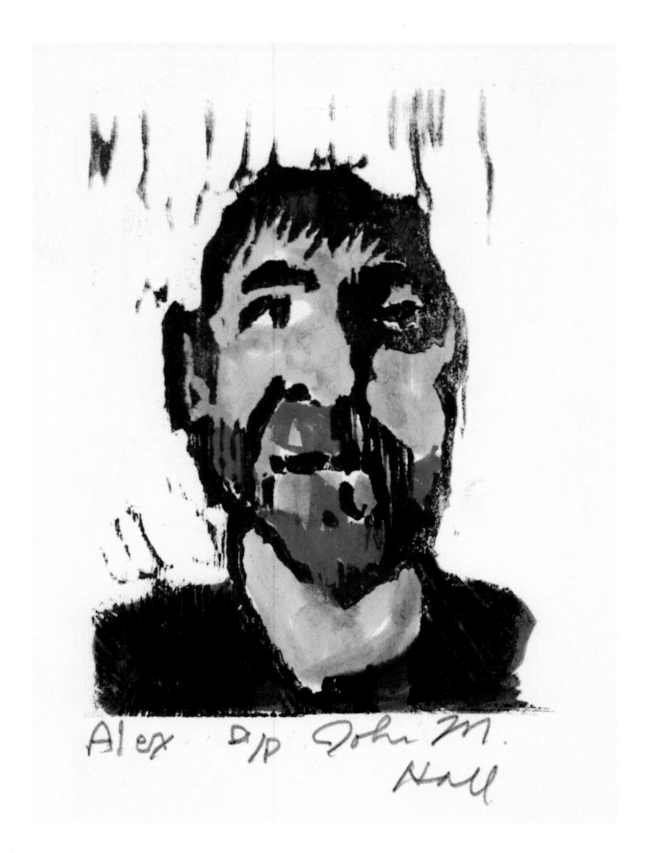

Alex, 1991. Watercolor woodcut, 6 x 4½ in.

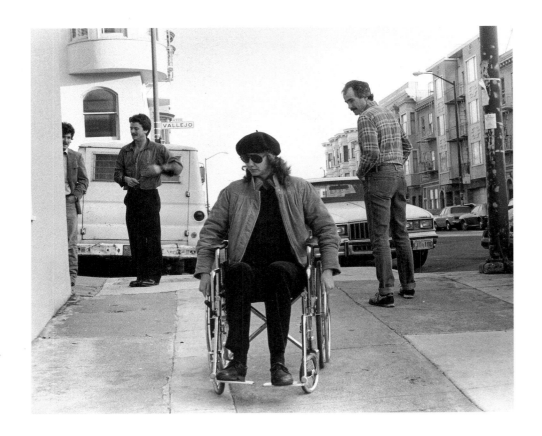

Angelina M. A. Hekking

San Francisco, California

"Over years a mutual respect developed that allowed me to see their character and spirit and capture it on film."

Angelina Hekking, a native of Holland, was diagnosed with MS at twenty-one years of age. Five years later, she moved to San Francisco to study photography. After a serious exacerbation, her physical limitations led her to experiment with self-portraits. During a recovery period, she started to study *t'ai chi* in Washington Square Park, where she photographed homeless people. Her self-portraits were published, along with her journal writings, in *Seeds of Light—Images of Healing* (Angel Publishing, San Francisco, 1991). Her photographs of the homeless have been exhibited internationally.

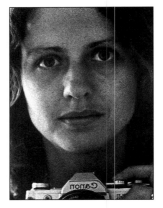

Another Relapse I Feel Devasted (Self-Portrait), 1984. Black-and-white photograph, 16 x 20 in.

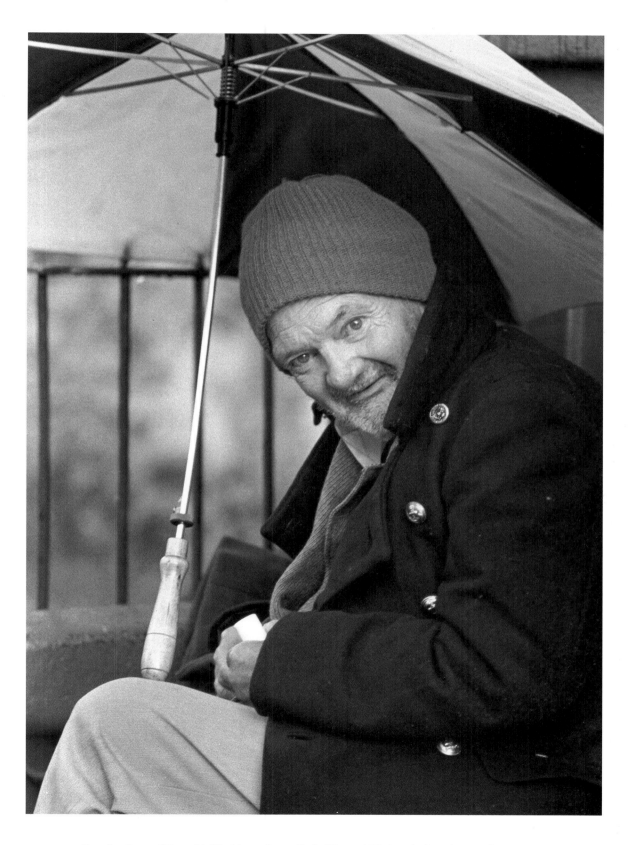

Homeless Person, "Homer" in Washington Square Park, S.F., 1986. Black-and-white photograph, 20 x 16 in.

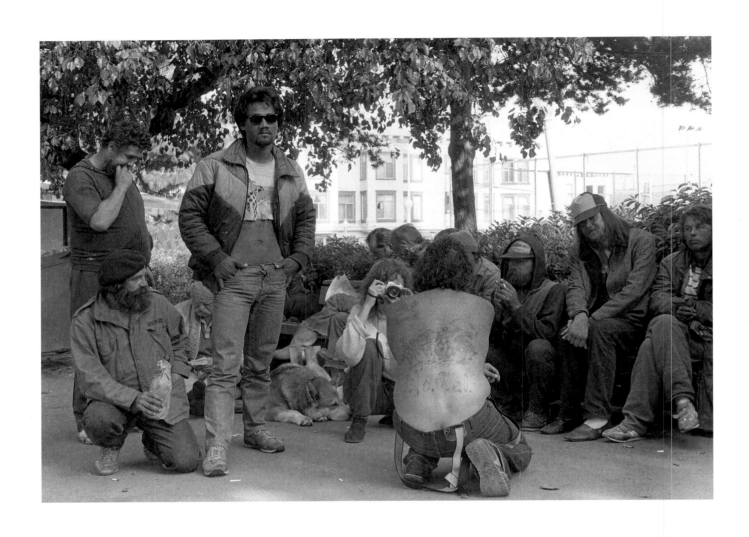

Homeless People in Washington Square Park, S.F. (Self-Portrait), 1986. Black and-white photograph, 16 x 20 in.
(The picture Hekking is taking in this photograph appears on the next page.)

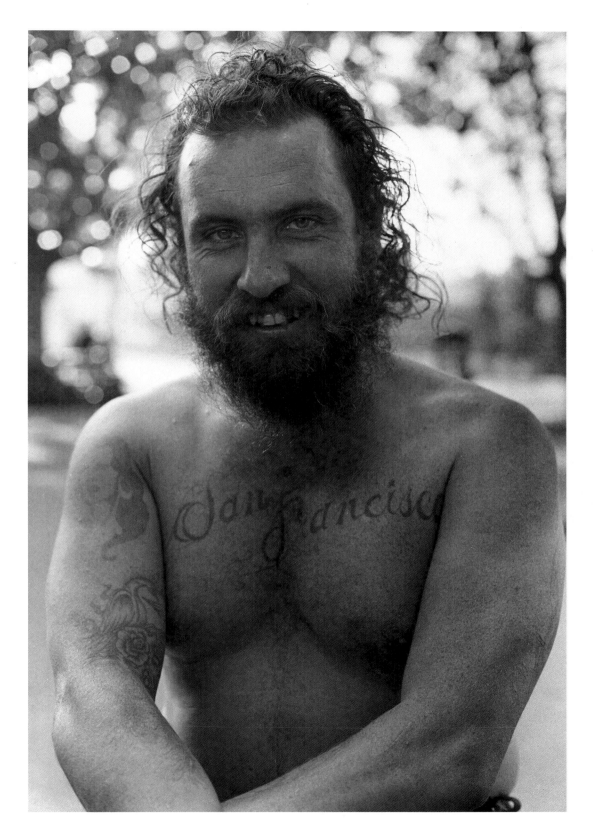

Homeless Person, "Tim" in Washington Square Park, S.F., 1986. Black-and-white photograph, 20 x 16 in.

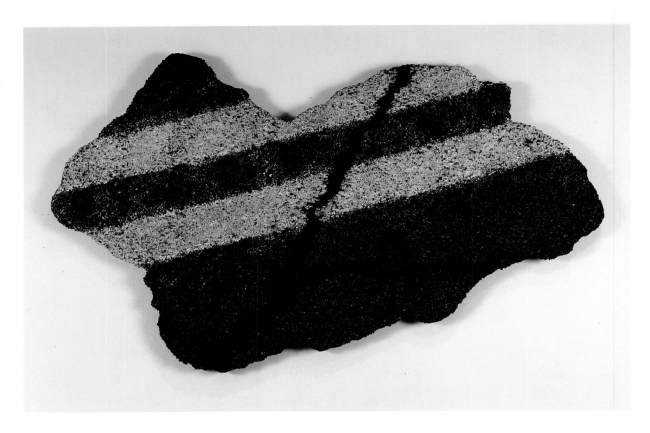

Thomas W. Hollender

Nutrioso, Arizona

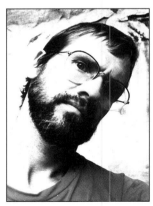

"My roadwork paintings are fractured representations of our consuming society."

Born in New York in 1954, Thomas Hollender moved west to study art and photography at the University of Arizona in Tucson. He remained in Arizona, where he became certified as an art teacher and librarian. Presently active as a sculptor, painter and photographer, Hollender has taught students in grade school through college and is currently a middle-school librarian. He has written and illustrated several children's picture books, for which he is seeking a publisher. Hollender was diagnosed with MS in 1987.

Untitled, 1992. Mixed media, 30 x 42 in.

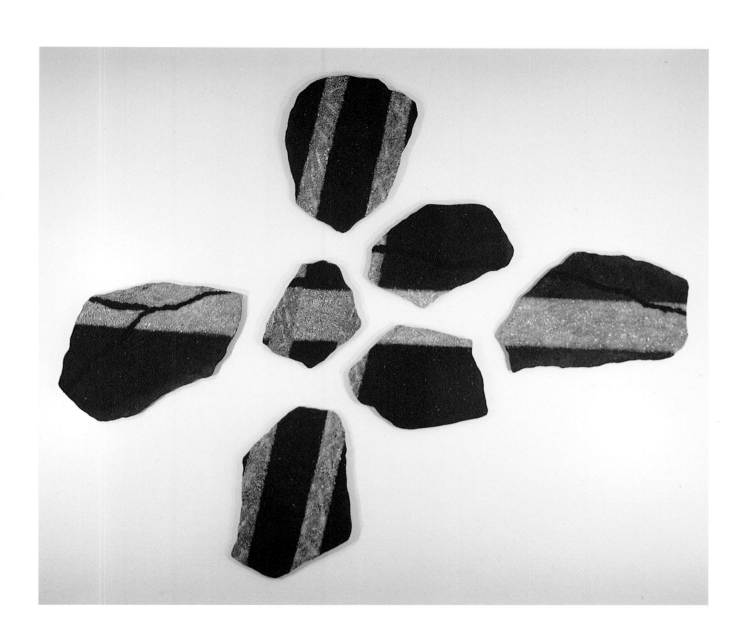

Cinder Pit #1, 1990. Mixed media on masonite, 96 x 120 in.

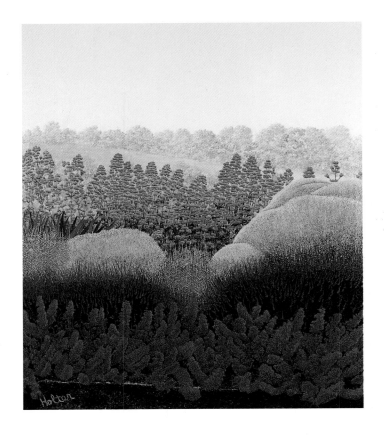

Robert Otis Holter

Scotts Valley, California

"A celebration of light—this is my goal when I paint."

After receiving a B.F.A. degree from San Jose State University in 1971, Robert Holter started a small graphic arts business specializing in fine pen-and-ink drawings. In 1979, he experienced severe hand cramps and changed his career to landscaping. Over the next six years, however, additional symptoms of what would eventually be diagnosed as MS—vision problems and fatigue—became obstacles. After giving up art altogether, Holter saw the 1991–1992 Project Rembrandt exhibit in San Francisco. Inspired by the determination of those artists, he started to paint again full time.

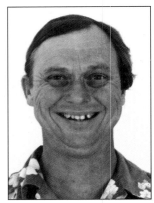

Kiss Me Quick in the Morning Mist, 1992. Acrylic on canvas, 48⅛ x 41⅛ in.

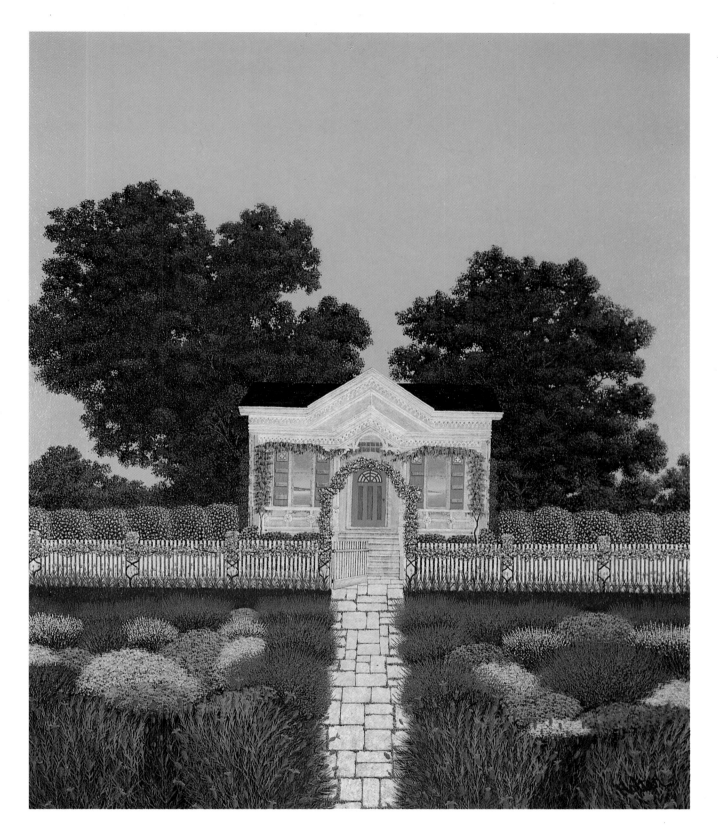

Portrait of a Victorian Lady, 1992. Acrylic on canvas, 61⅜ x 51 in.

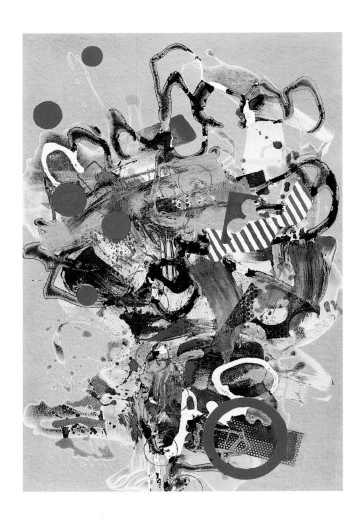

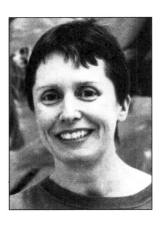

"My aim is to communicate directly with the emotions without . . . reproducing an object, to create order out of chaos, music out of noise."

Carol Hunt

Southampton, New York

Math and physics—subjects she taught for five years—as well as music and the "Far Eastern concept of negative space" all infuse Carol Hunt's paintings and monotypes with a freedom that took her many years to attain. She works on a very large scale, in defiance of her MS, with which she was diagnosed in 1972. Hunt has designed stage sets for the Anne Mackesey Dance Group. Her prize-winning art is represented by galleries in New York City and Southampton, New York, and she exhibits widely. Her paintings and prints are found in many major public and private collections.

Improvisation (M4J2), 1992. Monotype, 53¼ x 38⅛ in.

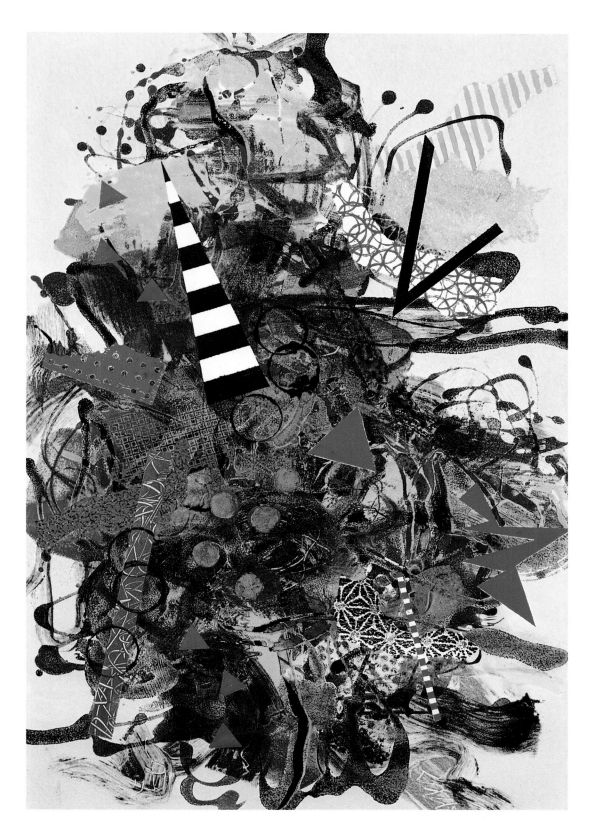

Improvisation (M4F2), 1992. Monotype, 36 x 24 in.

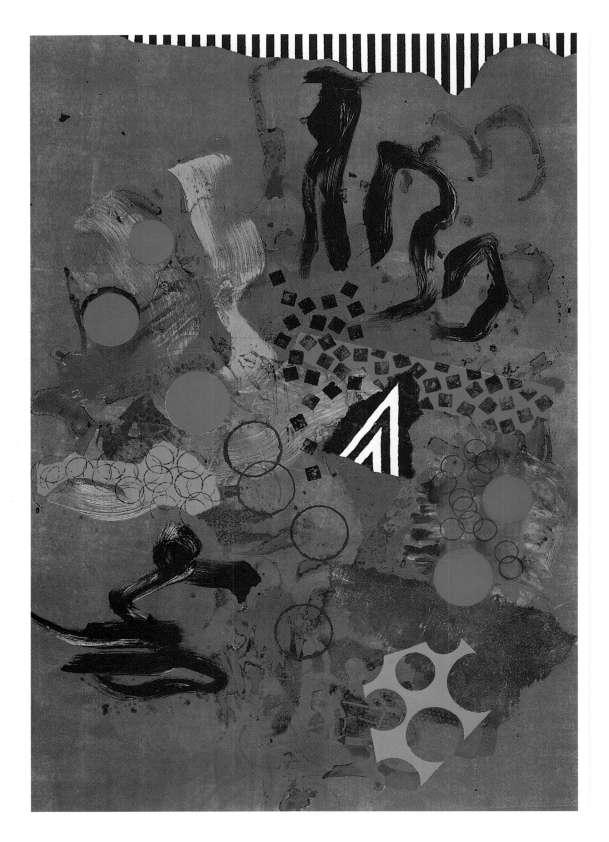

Improvisation (M4J3), 1992. Monotype, 53¼ x 38⅛ in.

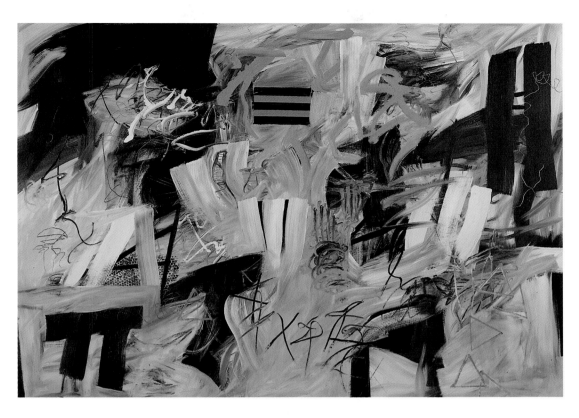

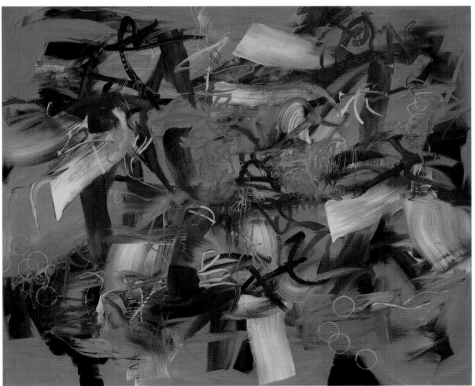

Remembered Suns, 1991. Oil on canvas, 66 x 90 in. (top) *Zapote,* 1992. Oil on canvas, 60 x 72 in. (bottom)

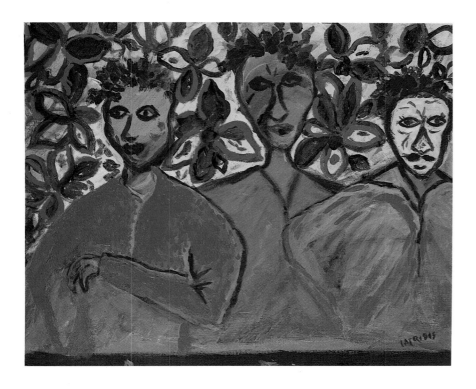

James Iatridis

Tenafly, New Jersey

"It's not my purpose to make pretty pictures....
My paintings are a visual barometer of [our]
times...and represent a very personal view."

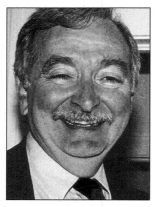

After receiving a business degree from New York University in 1959, James Iatridis was drafted into the army and stationed in Washington, D.C. He then began painting lessons at the Corcoran School of Art. Upon his return to civilian life, Iatridis attended Pratt Institute in Brooklyn for architectural design, leading to a career at the renowned design firms Knoll Associates and Stendig, Inc. Diagnosed with MS in 1978, he retired in 1985 because of fatigue. At home, he resumed painting after a thirty-year respite. In 1991 he began exhibiting his work.

Travelers, 1990. Acrylic on canvas, 20 x 24 in.

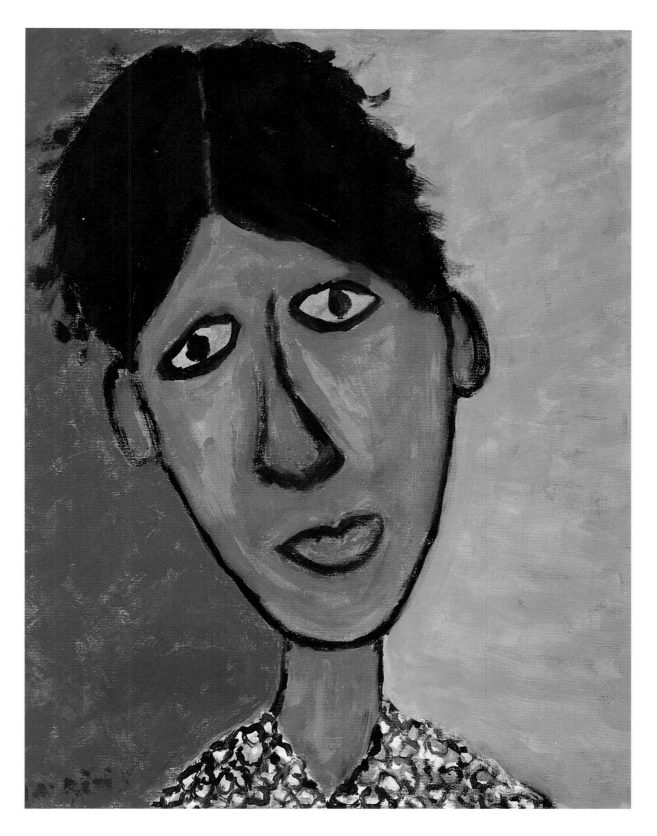

Irene I, 1990. Acrylic on canvas, 20 x 16 in.

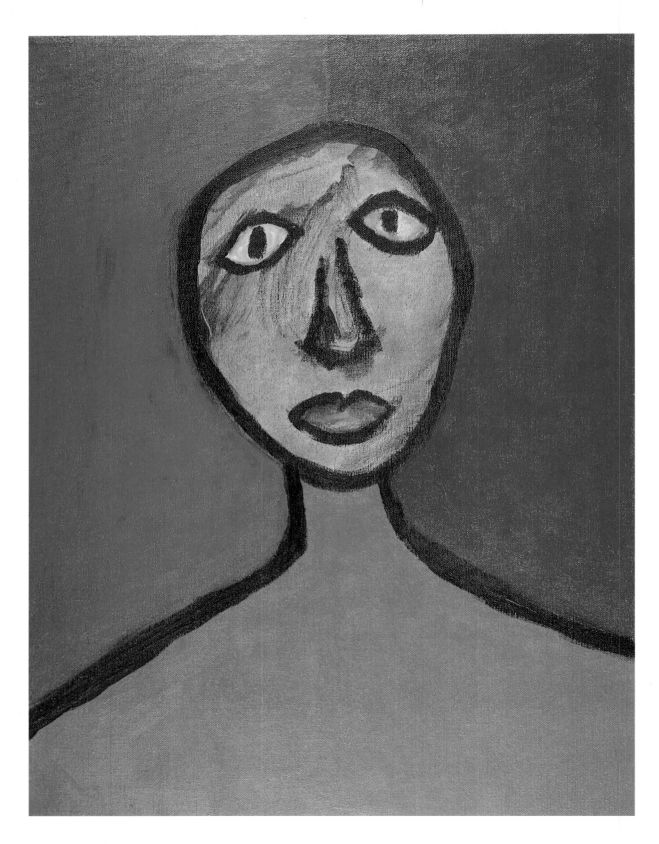

Woman #1, 1991. Acrylic on canvas, 24 x 18 in.

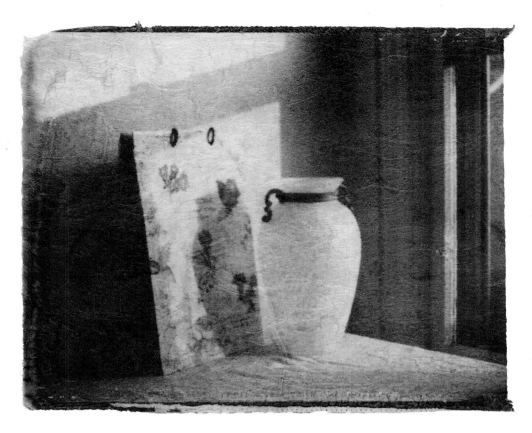

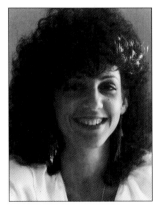

"Some things force us to see with a clarity of vision, in spite of what we may dream of seeing. MS has served to intensify [my] clarity."

Dina Kawer

Huntington Woods, Michigan

In 1979, Dina Kawer was diagnosed at age twenty-two with MS. That year she received a B.F.A. degree in photography from Wayne State University, where she also had studied painting and printmaking. Kawer asserts that as an artist and mother of two children, "MS is simply the least of that which defines me." Her delicate still-lifes are created through a unique process she has named "Polaroid Transfer Printing." She peels away the Polaroid film negative and applies it directly to special paper, custom-made exclusively for her by a Japanese craftsman. Her work is found in the Detroit Institute of Arts and other art institutions internationally.

Roman Vessel, 1992. Polaroid transfer image on Japanese kozo paper, 3¼ x 4¼ in.

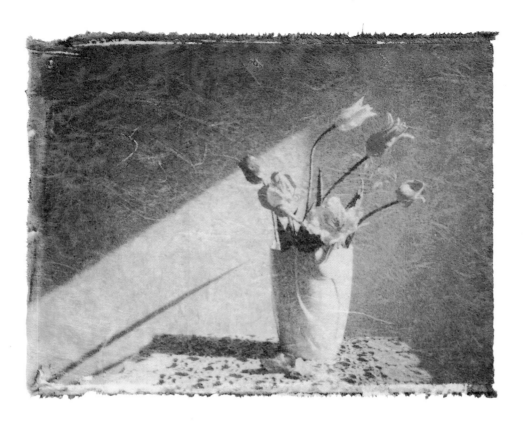

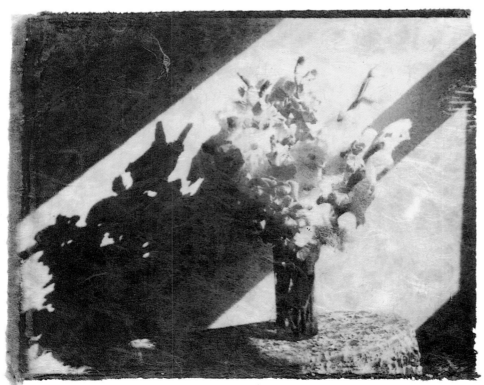

Tulips II, 1992. Polaroid transfer image on Japanese kozo paper, 3¼ x 4¼ in. (top)
Gladiolus, 1992. Polaroid transfer image on Japanese kozo paper, 3¼ x 4¼ in. (bottom)

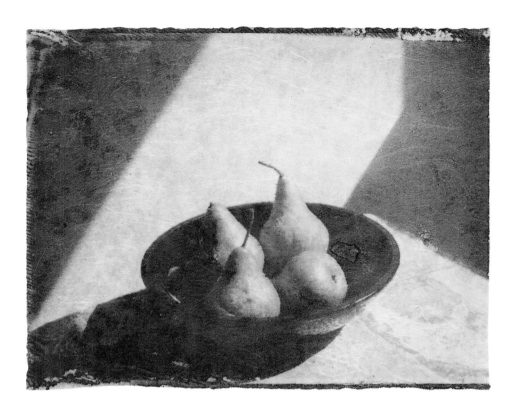

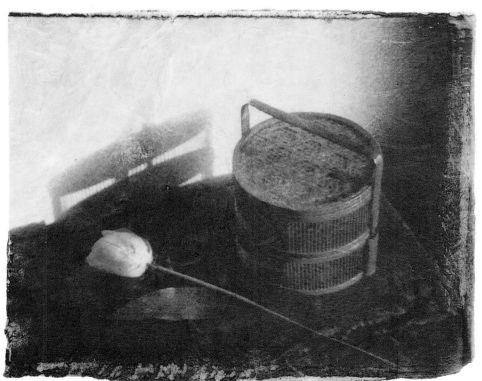

Four Pears, 1992. Polaroid transfer image on Japanese kozo paper, 3¼ x 4¼ in. (top)
Chinese Lacquer, 1992. Polaroid transfer image on Japanese kozo paper, 3¼ x 4¼ in. (bottom)

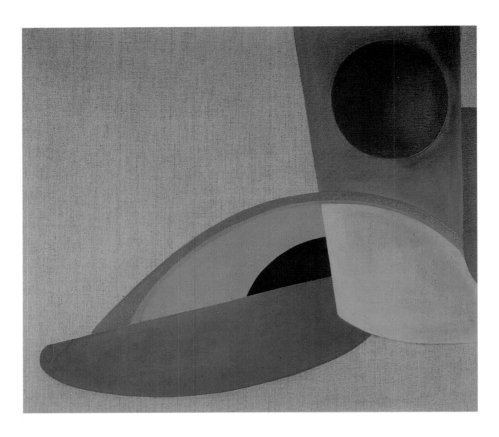

Frieda King

Long Beach, California

"The kaleidoscope of shapes and colors that surround me daily is mirrored in my abstracts."

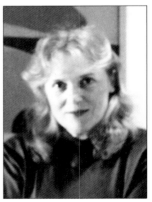

Frieda King was awarded an art scholarship by the Carnegie Institute in Oakland, Pennsylvania, when she was only eleven years old. She continued her education, earning a B.F.A. degree at California State University, Long Beach, in drawing and painting. King is also a photographer and sculptor. Diagnosed with MS in 1967, the disease has had a recent impact on King's art. "I can't hold my brushes the way I used to, so I have decided to switch to sculpture. Luckily, in counterbalance, my artistic perception continues to improve as I get older." She exhibits throughout southern California.

Green Moon, 1992. Oil on canvas, 28 x 32¼ in.

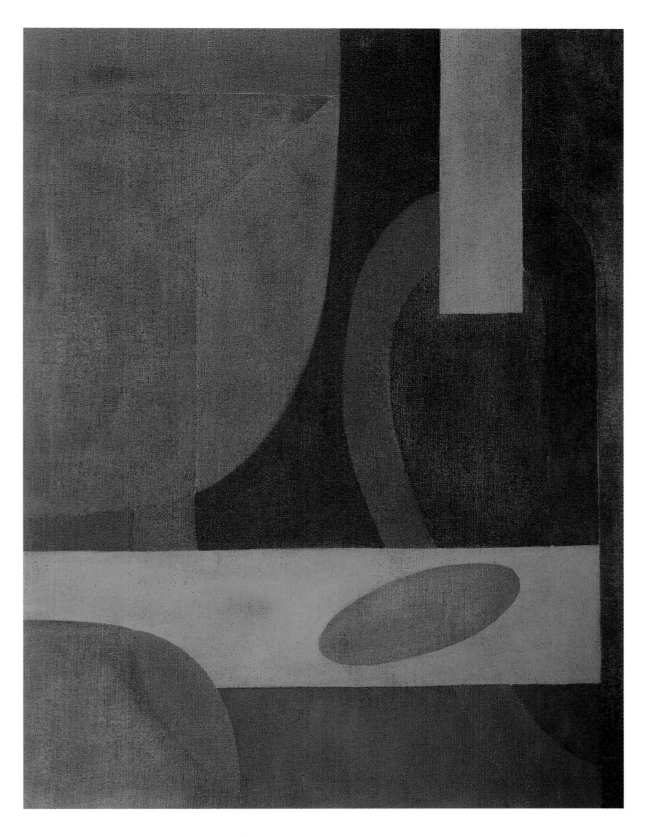

Reflections, 1990. Oil on canvas, 33 x 24 in.

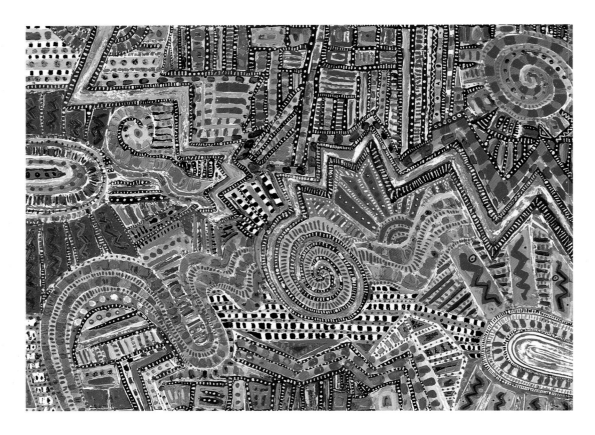

Rona Ginn Klein

Abington, Pennsylvania

"Painting [in all of its permutations] is the only opportunity that a mere mortal has to create a universe."

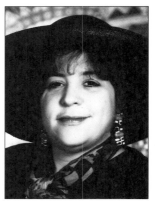

Rona Ginn Klein says that she is most influenced by the powerful interplay between color, shape and line that is a distinctive trait of African, pre-Columbian and Aboriginal art. She aims to achieve that power in her own art, which "includes but is not limited to" paintings, prints, collages, fiber pieces and poems (she is a published poet). Klein holds degrees in education from Temple University, Philadelphia, and she worked for the Philadelphia school system until 1987, when MS curtailed that facet of her career. Klein's art is found in public and private collections internationally.

Self Portrait IV Revisited, 1993. Mixed media, 22 x 30 in.

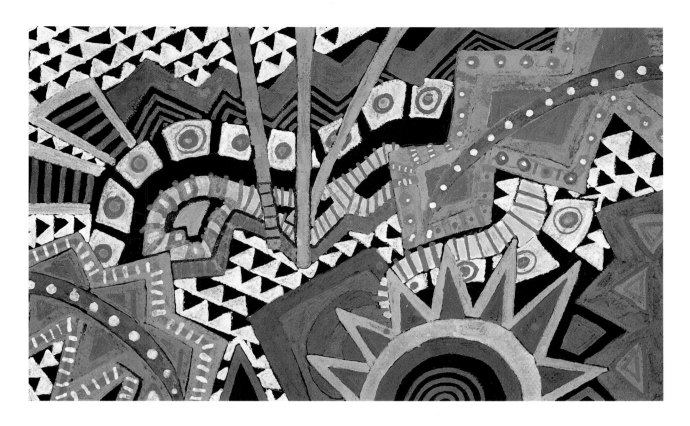

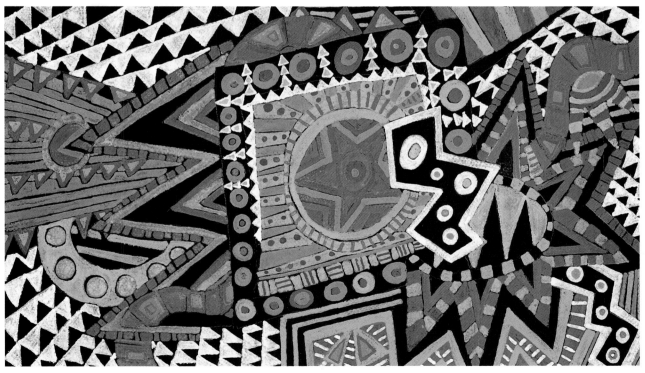

Synergy I, 1992. Color laser print, 17 x 23 in. (top) *Synergy II,* 1992. Color laser print, 17 x 23 in. (bottom)

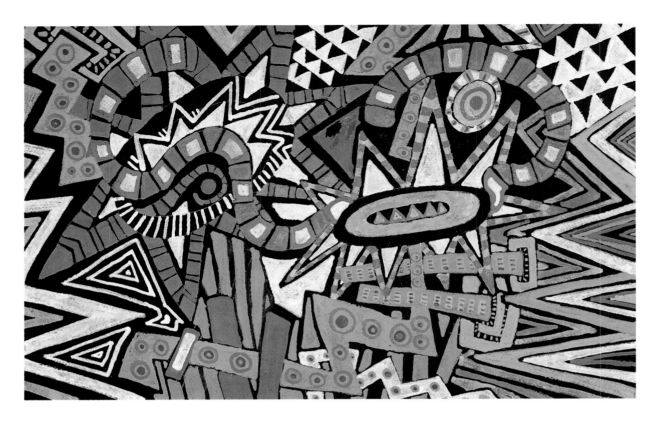

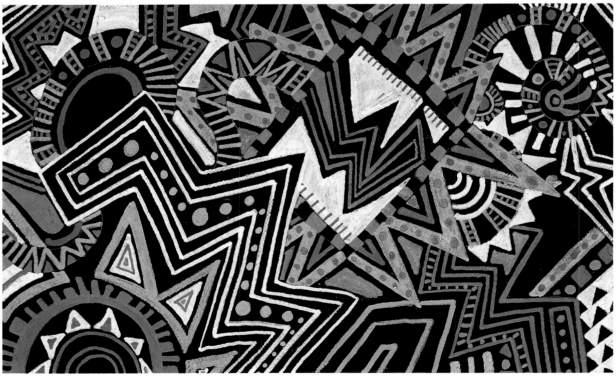

Synergy III, 1992. Color laser print, 17 x 23 in. (top) *Synergy IV,* 1992. Color laser print, 17 x 23 in. (bottom)

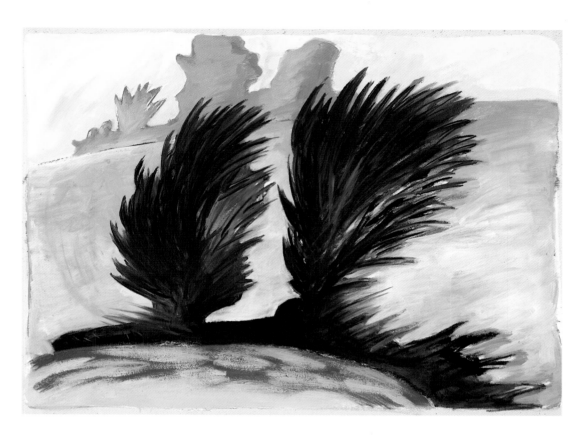

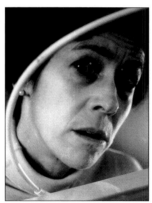

"If I respect my body and let it lie down when it wants to, then the ideas come."

"I have to sit down a good deal. I am forced to . . . spend more time . . . working with ideas. I started painting again. I got back to basics." These are some of the ways video/performance/fine artist Jessie Jane Lewis has recently accommodated MS when creating art. Lewis, diagnosed with the disease fifteen years ago, has performed or shown work at Creative Time's Art in the Anchorage, Brooklyn; the Whitney Museum of American Art; Nexus and The Painted Bride Art Center, Philadelphia, among other museums and organizations. Lewis is also a part-time recreation specialist for the elderly.

Jessie Jane Lewis

Philadelphia, Pennsylvania

Catskill Landscape, 1988. Oil on paper, 25½ x 33 in.

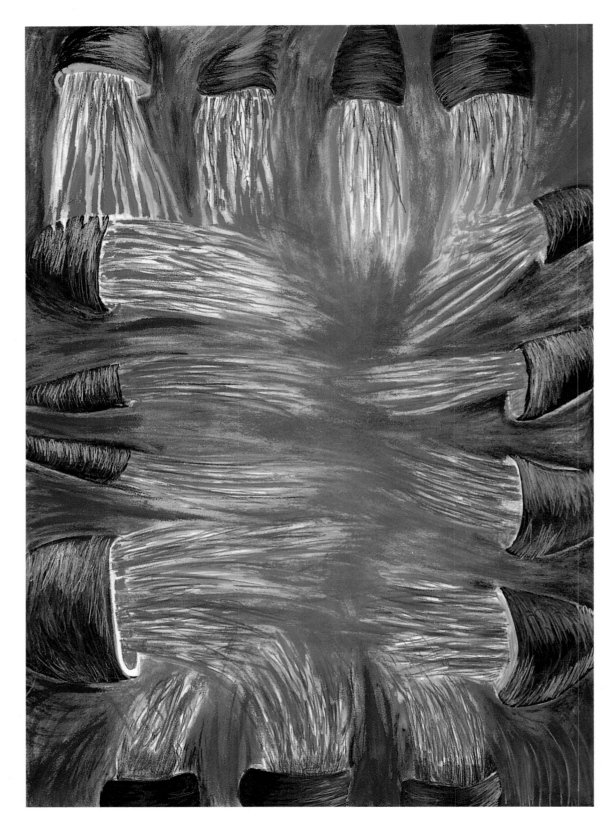

Electrical Circuits, 1989. Pastel and graphite on paper, 46½ x 34 in.

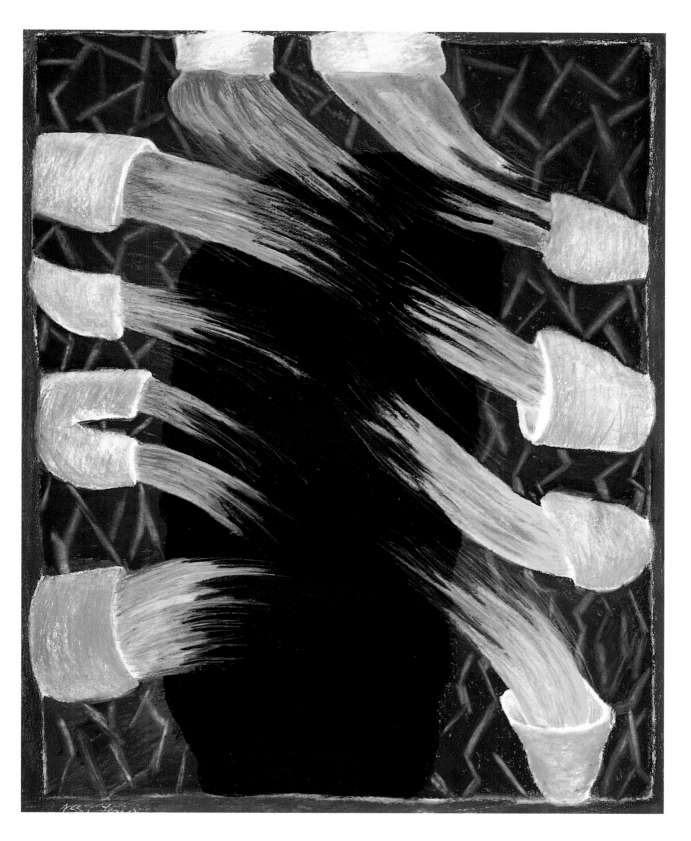

Pink Flesh Contacts, 1989. Pastel and graphite on paper, 44⅜ x 36½ in.

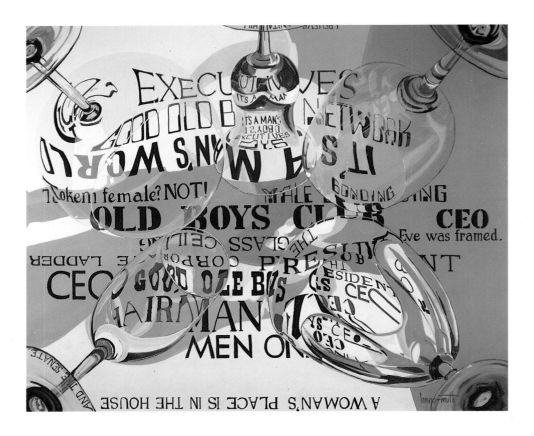

Linda L. Longo-Muth

Valley Cottage, New York

"My work concentrates on the movement, reflection and penetration of light through glass."

Linda Longo-Muth perceives that the movement of light penetrating glass, her chosen subject, is symbolic of the unexpected direction her life has taken. Longo-Muth's art studies brought her to Italy and France, among other places. In 1987, MS ended her teaching career but liberated her to become a full-time artist. Longo-Muth's award-winning paintings now hang in important corporate and private collections nationwide, and she exhibits extensively. She was a featured speaker at The Museum of Modern Art's "Women Artists Disabled" symposium.

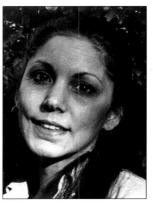

The Glass Ceiling, 1992. Acrylic on canvas, 41 x 49 in.

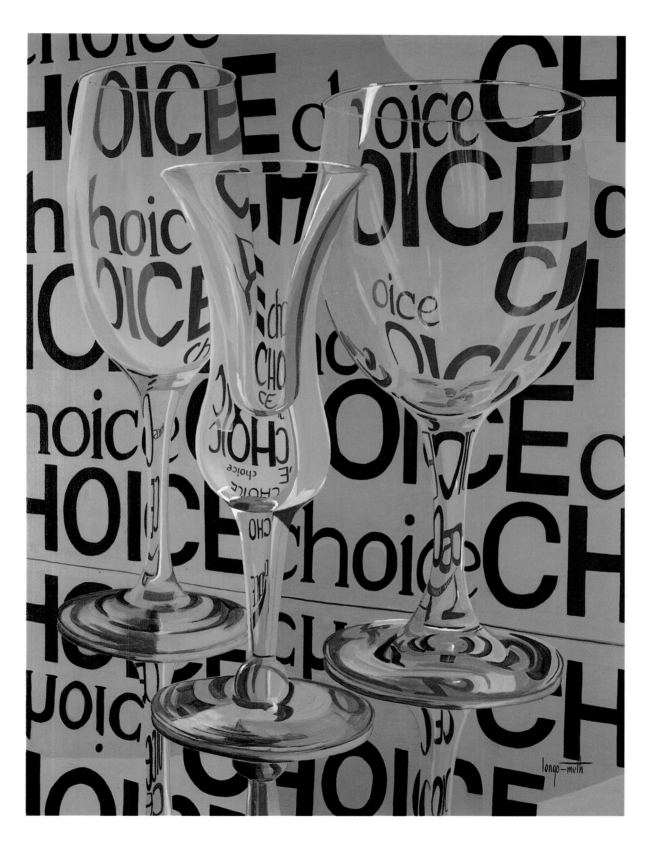

It's Your Choice, 1992. Acrylic on canvas, 49 x 37 in. Private collection.

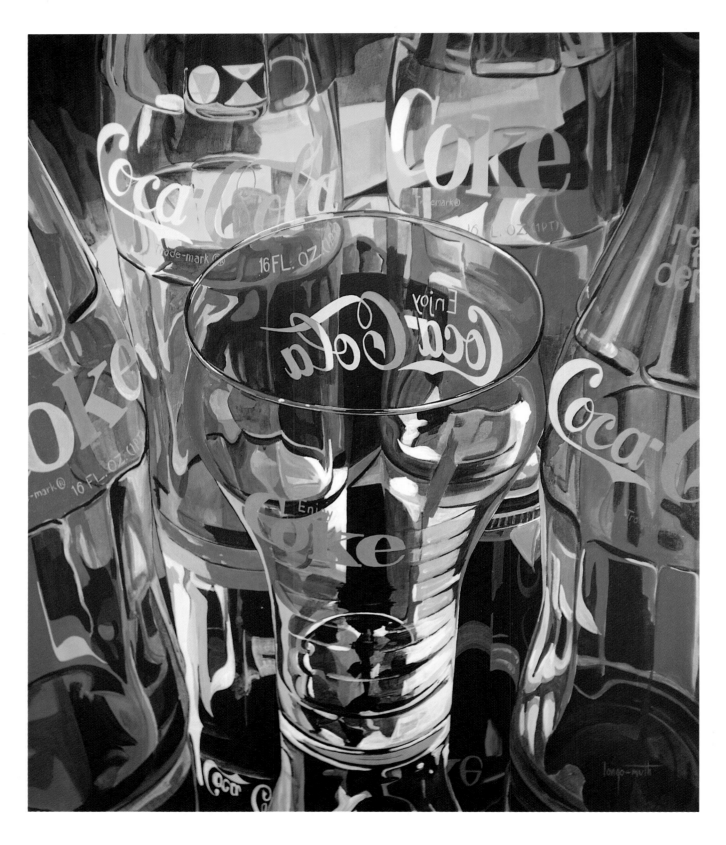

The Glass of '92, 1991. Acrylic on canvas, 49 x 41 in.

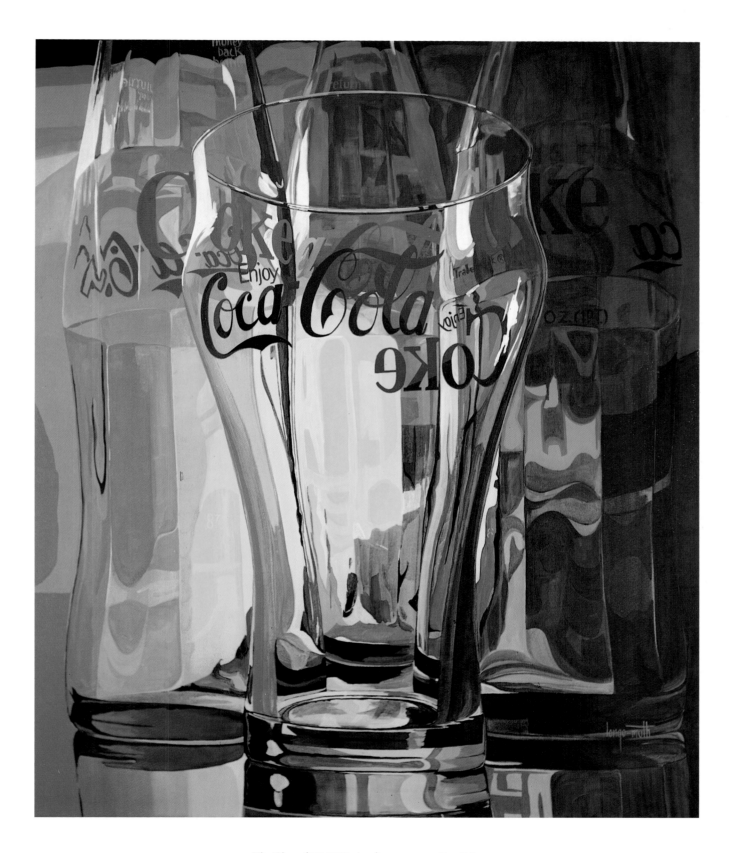

The Glass of '93, 1992. Acrylic on canvas, 49 x 41 in.

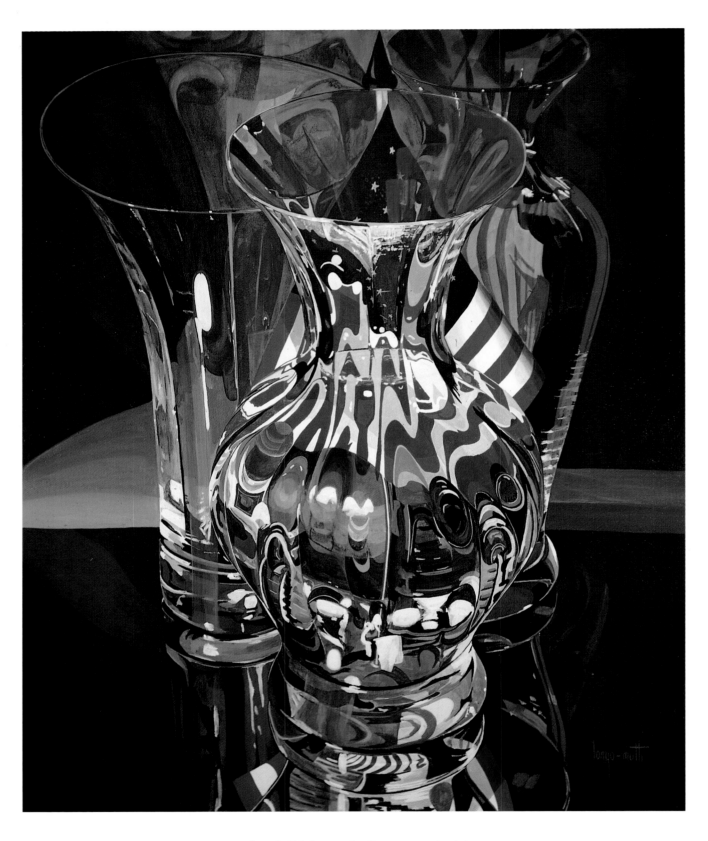

Made in the U.S.A., 1991. Acrylic on canvas, 49 x 41 in.

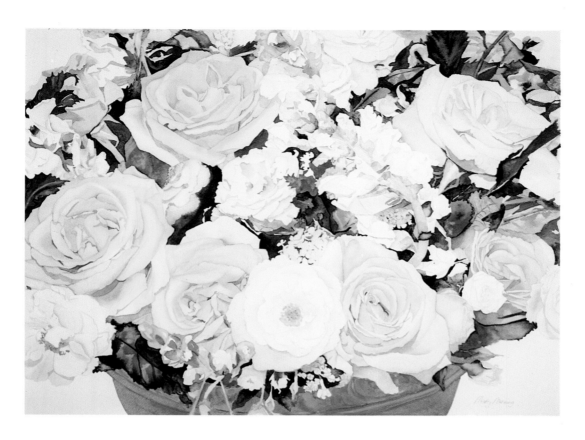

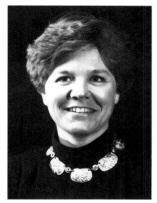

"I concern myself with nature's objects seen closely...searching for 'the true and the beautiful.'"

Marty Manning

Fairfax, Virginia

Marty Manning began her art career creating batiks on rice paper, a technique she developed. Although she recalls experiencing her first MS symptoms in 1969, it wasn't until 1981 that she was diagnosed, when she experienced a debilitating exacerbation including serious vision problems and weakness. After a slow recuperation, Manning began to paint again, but changed her palette and perspective from dark brooding pieces to bright floral watercolors. Her work is exhibited nationally and is found in many corporate, public and private collections. It is also reproduced commercially.

Rose Bowl, 1990. Watercolor and gouache on paper, 22 x 30 in. Courtesy of Newmark Publishing USA.

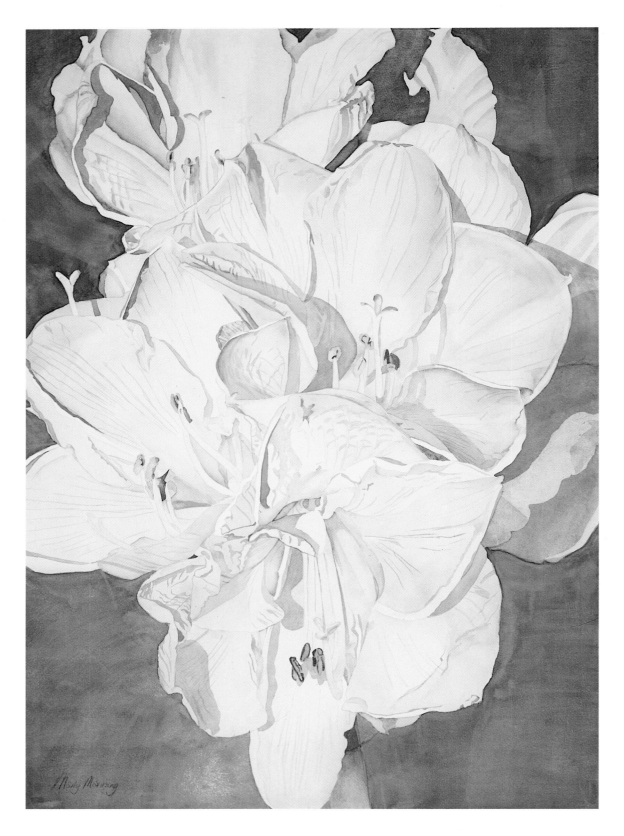

Amaryllis Snow White, 1990. Watercolor and gouache on paper, 48 x 36 in. Courtesy of Newmark Publishing USA.

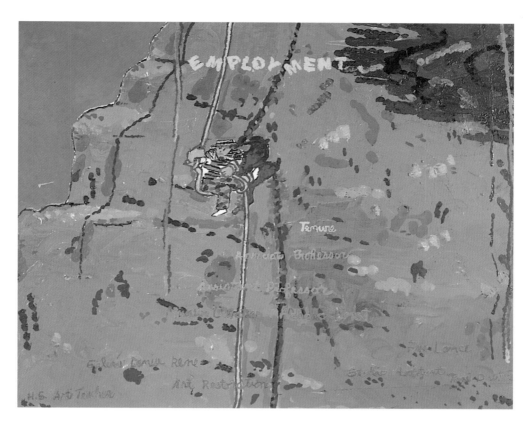

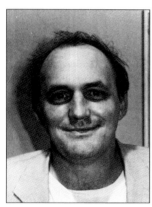

"I've never climbed real walls. These are symbolic walls—of employment and aging. The paintings show struggle, but also triumph."

Thomas Martin

New York, New York

Thomas Martin—diagnosed with MS in 1978—has found that the major effect the disease has on his art is to diminish the time he can stand in front of an easel. This, he says, makes him "depend less on manual facility and more on conceptual facility. My work is becoming more introspective." His work is also often autobiographical. Formerly a curator at the Museum of the American Indian, Heye Foundation, Martin is currently associate professor MAC/Arts Area at the New York Institute of Technology in Old Westbury.

Employment, 1989. Oil on canvas, 24 x 36 in.

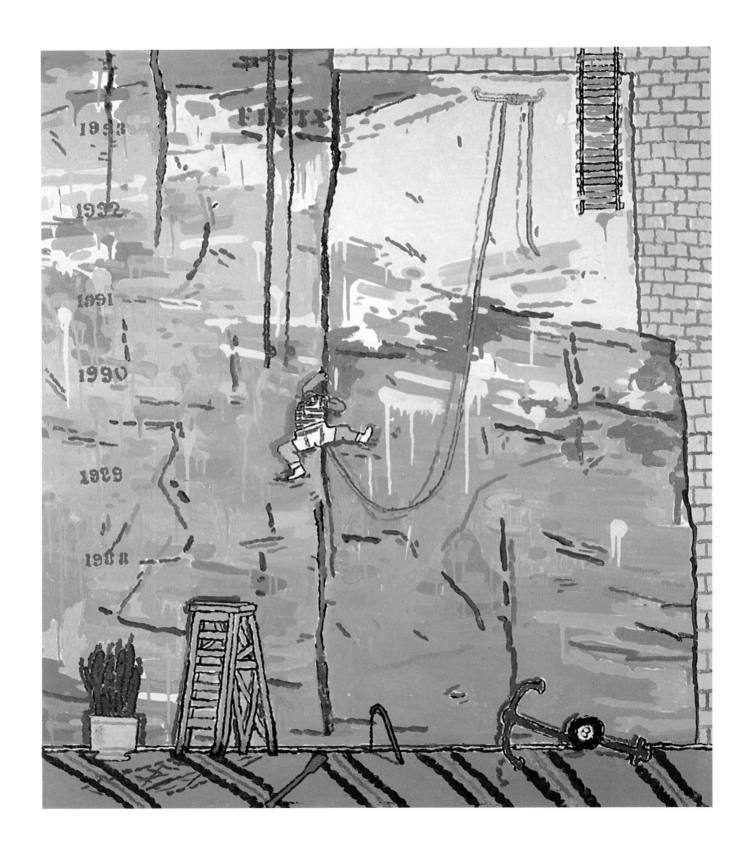

Ages 45 to 50, 1991. Oil on canvas, 60 x 48 in.

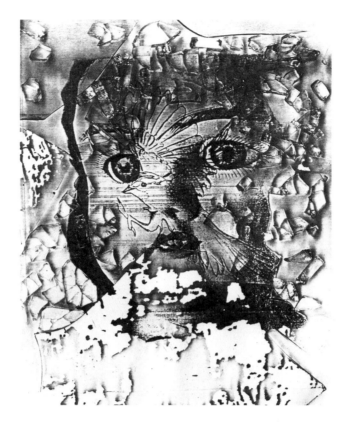

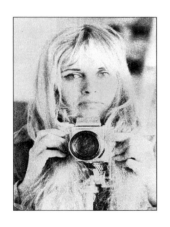

"I did [these photos] just after recovering from a frightening MS bout in which I lost my eyesight."

Ruby McLain is a self-taught photographer who received some darkroom technical training from Brig Cabe, a Washington, D.C., photojournalist. In 1974 she worked at The Fenn Studios in Paris with Gene Fenn, an international fashion photographer and filmmaker. McLain's photos have been exhibited at the Virginia Museum of Art in Richmond and the Corcoran Gallery of Art and Gallery K in Washington, D.C., among other galleries and institutions. Her work also has been published in newspapers and reproduced commercially. She is best known for her painting and sculpture, which she creates under the name Ruby Grady. McLain was diagnosed with MS in 1970.

Ruby McLain

Fort Washington, Maryland

Fragile, 1989. Black-and-white photograph, 20 x 16 in.

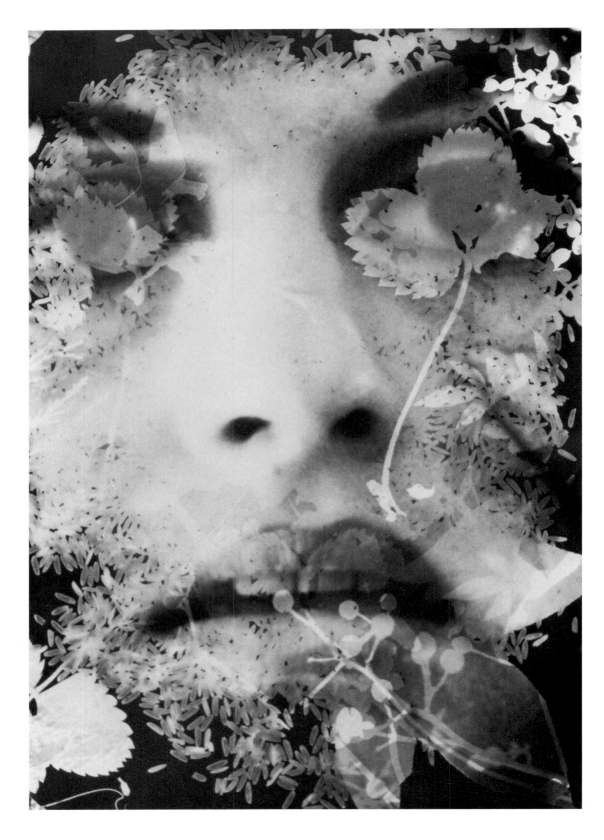

Senses, 1990. Black-and-white photograph, 28 x 22 in.

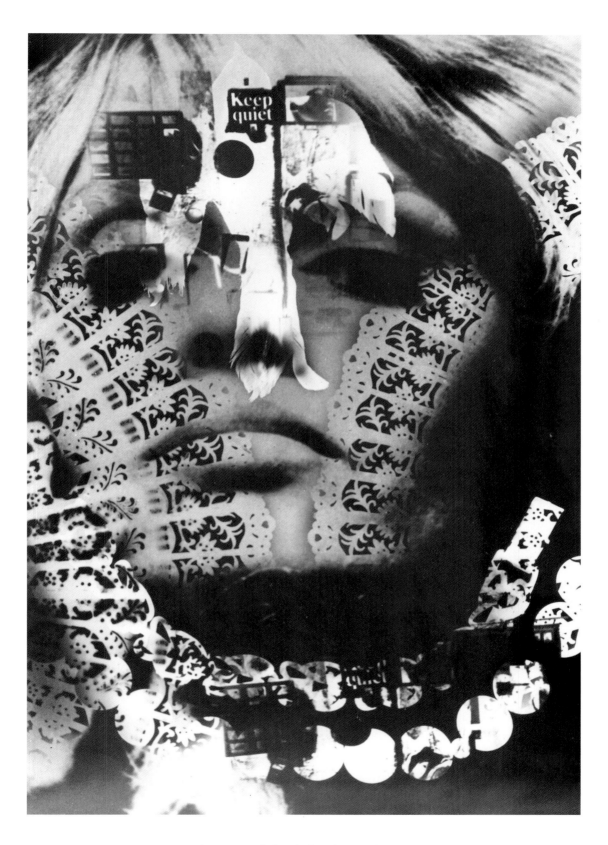

Keep Quiet, 1989. Black-and-white photograph, 20 x 16 in.

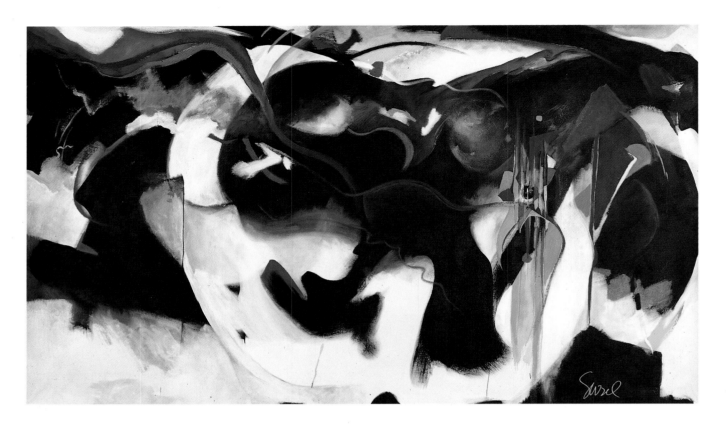

Surel Mitchell

Boise, Idaho

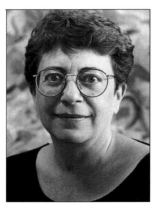

"Making art is an egocentric act. One does it in isolation. . . . Sharing work takes the isolation away and makes [it] universal."

Surel Mitchell uses color, texture, line, composition and movement to create what she describes as "inner-scapes"—the landscapes of her psyche. She was diagnosed with MS in 1984 after it had affected her vision, leaving her temporarily blind in one eye. Today, her most difficult symptom is extreme fatigue, which she accommodates by taking time off when it intensifies and painting as hard as she can when it subsides. Mitchell exhibits throughout the country, and her work is found in many corporate and private collections.

AE-6, 1991. Acrylic on unstretched canvas, 83 x 49 in.

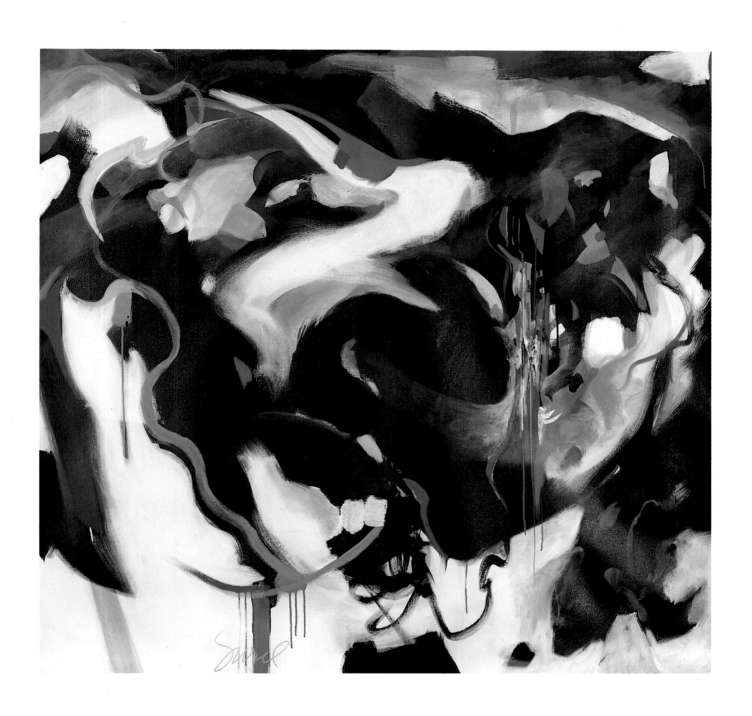

AE-5, 1991. Acrylic on unstretched canvas, 60 x 57 in.

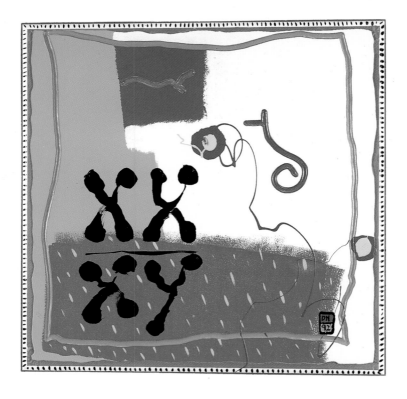

Debra Norby

Portland, Oregon

"I've always been interested in life forms. . . . I've now started focusing on those which are most basic."

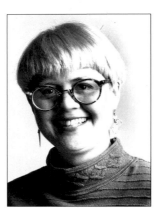

Debra Norby became a full-time ceramic sculptor in 1982, when MS ended her career in advertising as a graphic artist. While she continues to work primarily in clay, a recent donation of wood from the Louisiana-Pacific Corporation has sparked a new exploration in painting. Norby explains that her current work also addresses three-dimensionality: she uses a router to make lines in the wood "for added depth and interest." She finds that she is starting to favor mixing mediums as well. Norby is represented by galleries across the country, and she exhibits extensively.

A Woman & A Man, 1992. House paint on wood, 24 x 24 in.

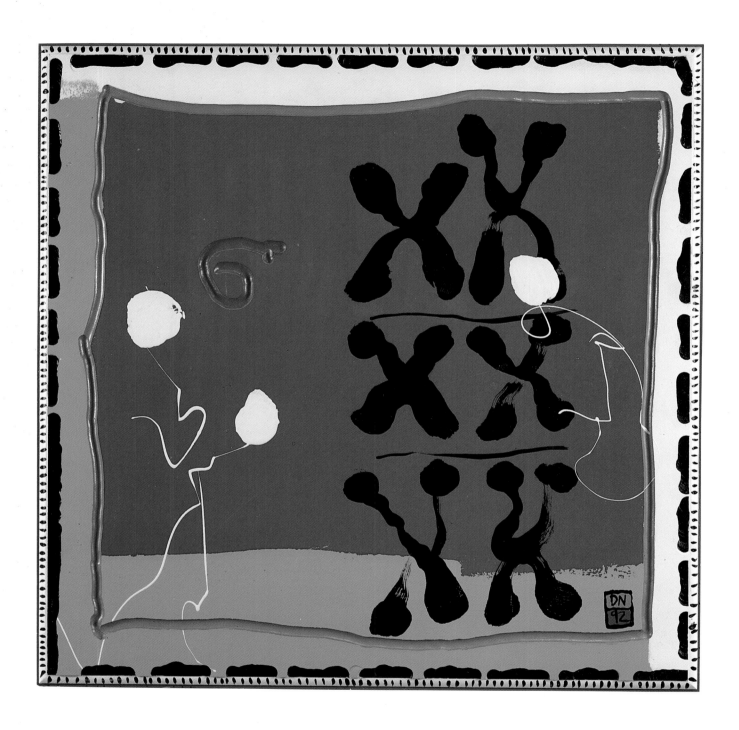

3 Women, 1992. House paint on wood, 24 x 24 in. Collection of Betsy Wolfston

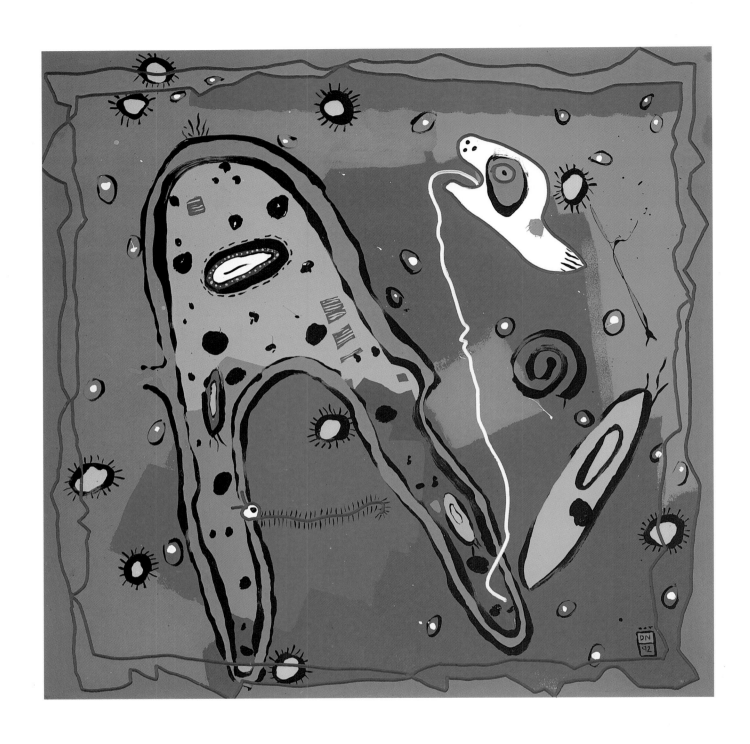

Pond Water 2, 1992. House paint on wood, 48 x 48 in.

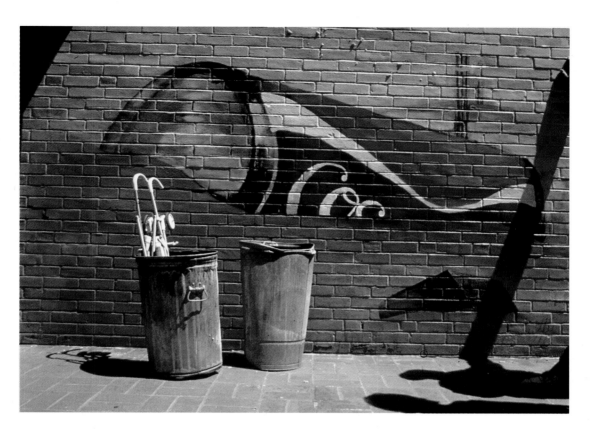

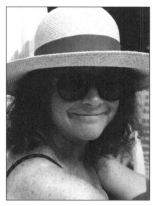

"Something or someone was juxtaposed . . . to introduce irony and tension."

Mary O'Hara Gregory studied editorial photography in college before working as a staff photographer for The SmithKline Beecham Corporation. She was diagnosed with MS in 1975 after losing her vision in one eye. Ten years later "the MS symptoms caught up with me. I left the corporate life to pursue my interest in 'fine art' photography and support this non-paying habit with freelance reportage photography work." O'Hara Gregory's photography is exhibited internationally.

Mary O'Hara Gregory

Philadelphia, Pennsylvania

A Classic, 1985. Color photograph, 20 x 24 in.

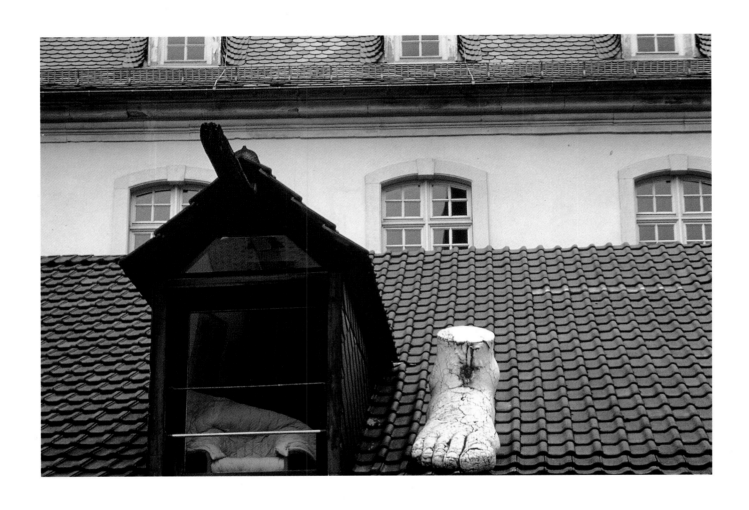

Just Put Your Foot Down, 1989. Color photograph, 20 x 24 in.

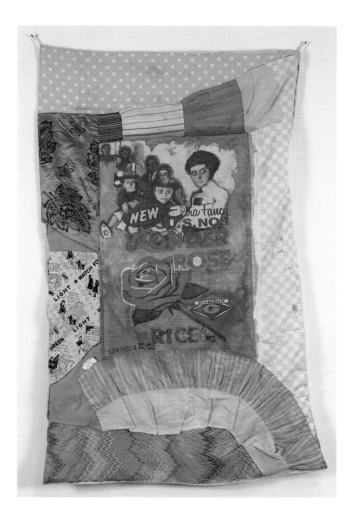

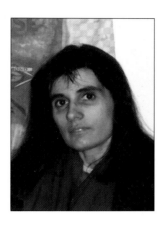

"I was looking for my face in the image of my grandmother, and this quilt grew as I assembled pieces from old skirts and found materials."

Jeana Sirabella was diagnosed with MS in 1977, the year she received a degree from the School of Visual Arts, New York City. She had attended SVA while working as the art director of an advertising agency, but soon after graduation MS fatigue symptoms forced her to leave. However, according to Sirabella, MS has not interfered with her creative spirit. Two of her interests—quilts and portraits—are combined in *Carmela II.* The quilt portrays Sirabella's grandmother and family before leaving Italy for Ellis Island. Sirabella's unique designs, which she describes as "windows on the wall," are exhibited nationally.

Jeana Sirabella

New York, New York

Carmela II, 1992. Oil on quilted fabric, 48 x 29 x 2 in.

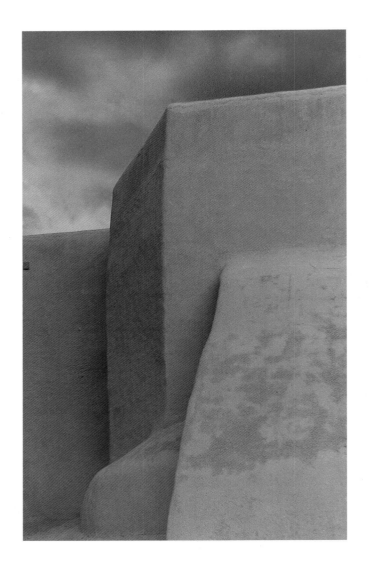

Karen G. Stone

Albuquerque, New Mexico

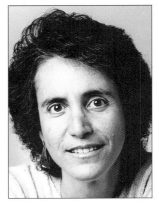

"New Mexico without adobe would be like . . . a temple without a shrine. I consecrate adobe. And photograph it as well."

After a twelve-year career as a commercial freelance photographer, MS gave new meaning to the importance of photography in Karen Stone's life. "I can share a great deal with others through this tool. My body may be slower; my faculties remain the same. The camera makes up the difference." Stone's photographs are infused with the light and history of New Mexico—a "magical" place, she says, that has affected her perceptions since youth. She is also a writer known for her very visual style. Stone finds it enriching to alternate between photography and writing. "One feeds into the other. There is no separation."

Ranchos de Taos, 1988. Color photograph, 20 x 16 in.

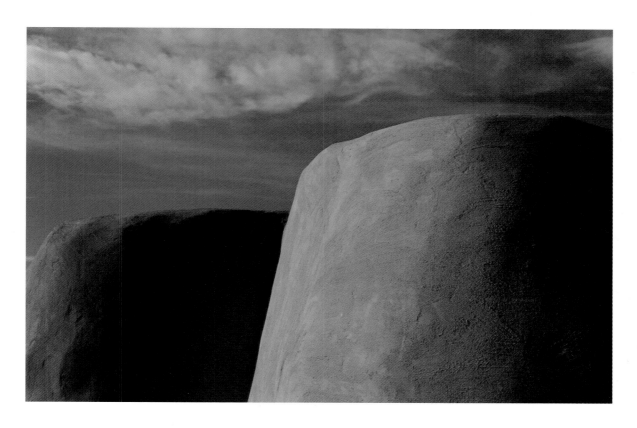

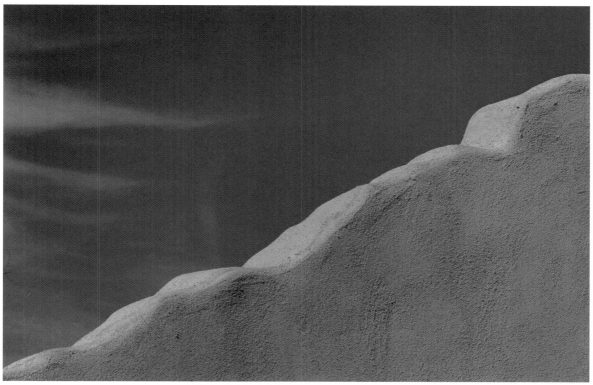

Kivas, Coronado Ruins, 1988. Color photograph, 16 x 20 in. (top) *Adobe Wall Detail,* 1989. Color photograph, 16 x 20 in. (bottom)

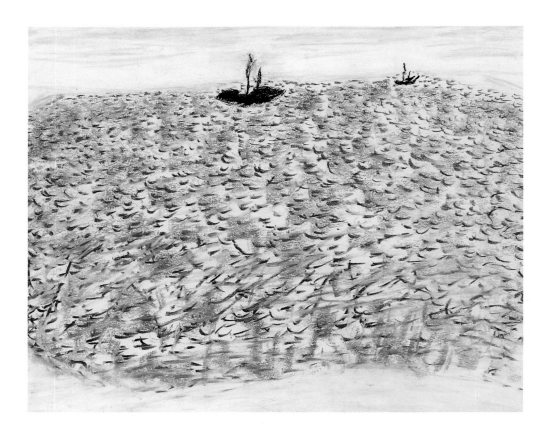

Charles Strouchler

New York, New York

"I'm stuck in my house a lot, so I take to dreaming.... If you close your eyes and concentrate, you can think of places...imaginary landscapes."

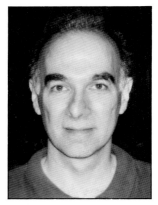

Charles Strouchler was born in the Bronx forty-eight years ago and has lived in New York City most of his life. Although he began painting with no formal instruction, he nevertheless was awarded a scholarship to the Provincetown Fine Arts Work Center in 1971. Ever since, he has worked as a professional photographer and painter. Strouchler has also been a cab driver, a screenplay writer, a box office manager at Carnegie Recital Hall and a still photographer for motion pictures. He developed MS seventeen years ago and has used a wheelchair since 1989.

Two Boats, 1989. Pastel on paper, 16½ x 18¾ in.

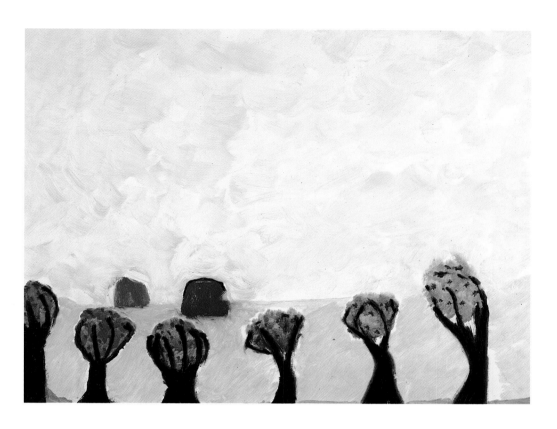

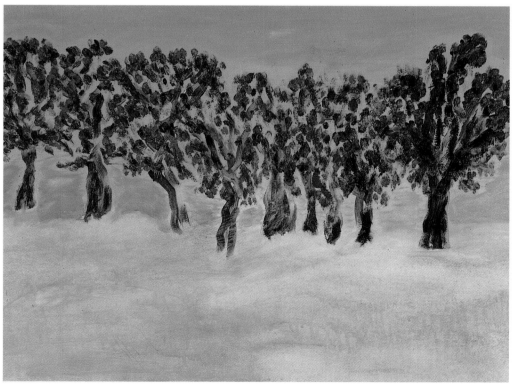

Two Barns, 1989. Oil on paper, 23½ x 29 in. (top) *The Trees,* 1990. Oil on paper, 22½ x 28¾ in. (bottom)

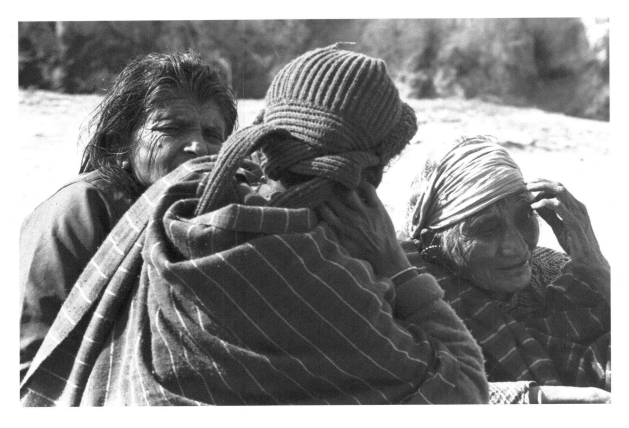

James Uhl

Kingston, Pennsylvania

"I feel what I see. . . . My photographs are the result of feelings, not ideas."

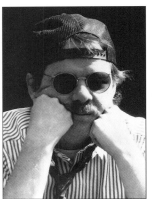

Jim Uhl is a self-taught freelance photographer who has always wanted to make the camera his career. While serving in the Coast Guard between high school and college, he first experimented with photography when stationed in Alaska. In 1971 he went on to complete his B.A. degree in political science with a minor in animal behavior. The camera, however, remained a deep interest. Uhl was diagnosed with MS in 1987. In 1989 he traveled to Nepal and India to photograph. Photography, he says, keeps him productive and is very therapeutic.

Old Friends, 1989. Black-and-white photograph, 11 x 14 in.

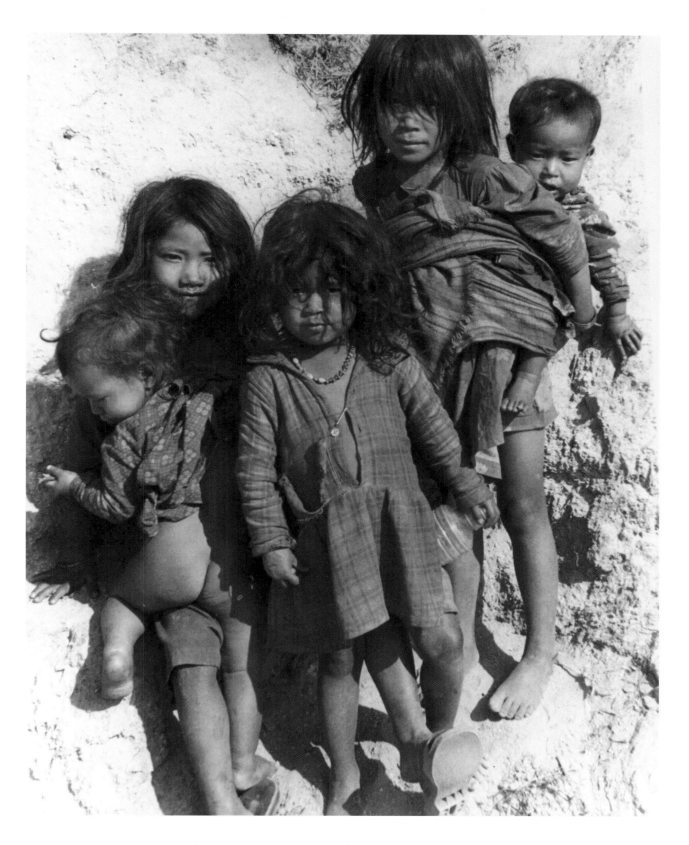

Nepalese Ragamuffins, 1989. Black-and-white photograph, 14 x 11 in.

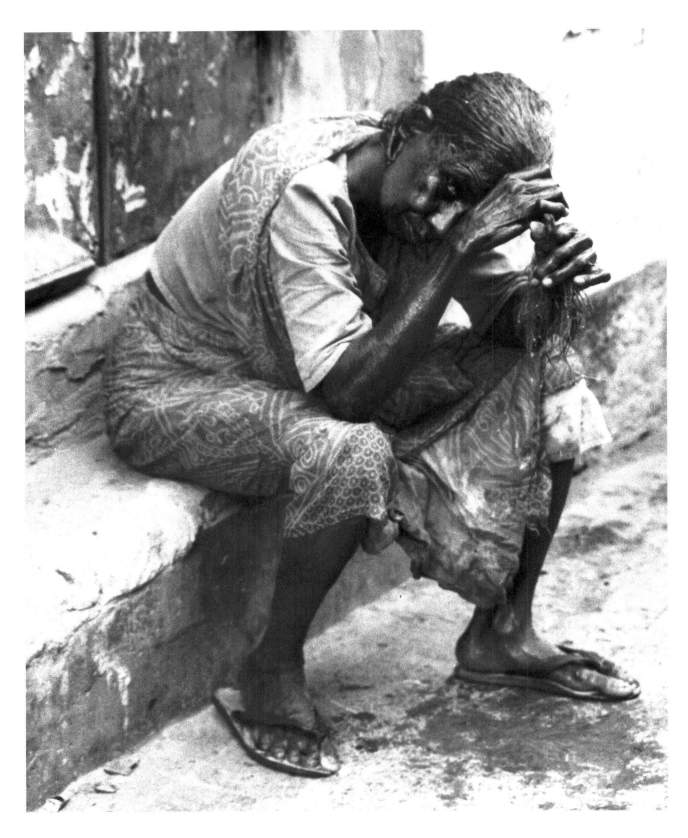

Hard Day's Night, 1989. Black-and-white photograph, 14 x 11 in.

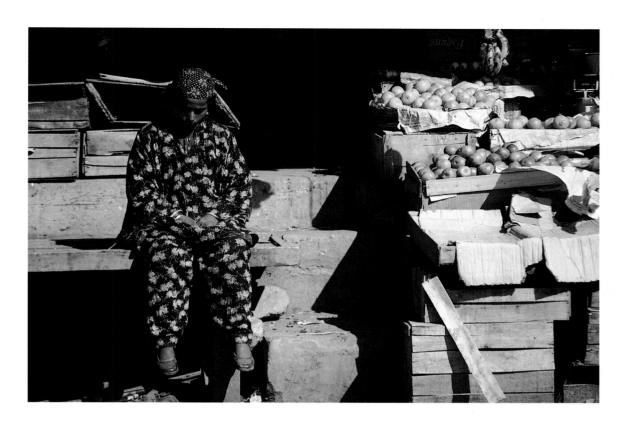

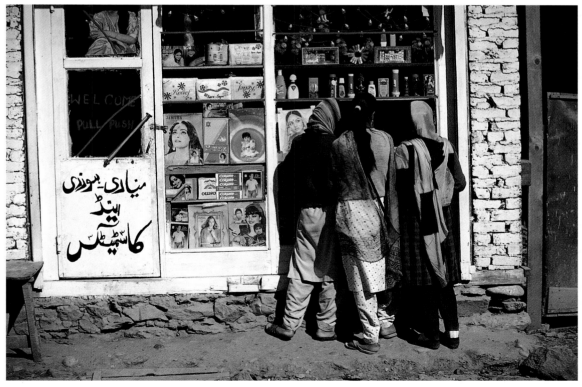

Modesty, 1989. Color photograph, 12 x 15 in. (top) *Dreaming,* 1989. Color photograph, 12 x 15 in. (bottom)

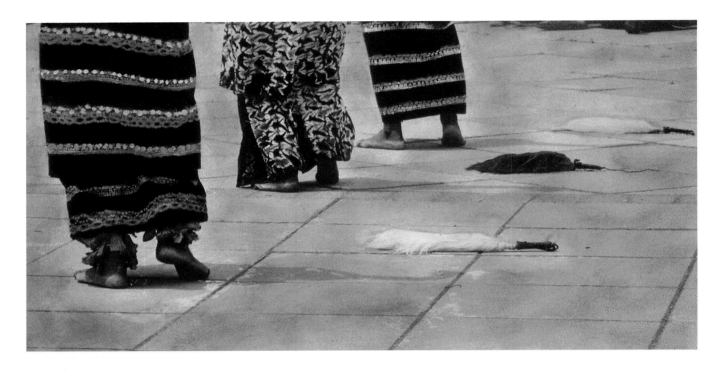

Lorna R. Warden

Richmond, Virginia

"I feel it's important not to take my surroundings for granted; to see beauty and know that there's more around every corner."

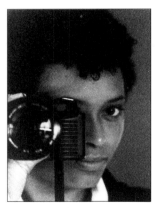

Lorna Warden was born in Richmond. After graduating from Howard University with a B.A. degree in communications she moved to New York City and worked for several years as a magazine publication coordinator. Although she traveled widely because of her job, Warden says it was not until she suddenly lost her vision and was subsequently diagnosed with MS in 1989 that she "began to appreciate the simple beauty of glances, skies and moments." Having since regained much of her sight, she is determined to see, photograph and paint as much of that beauty as she can for as long as possible.

Dancers, 1991. Hand-painted C-print photograph, 12½ x 16 in.

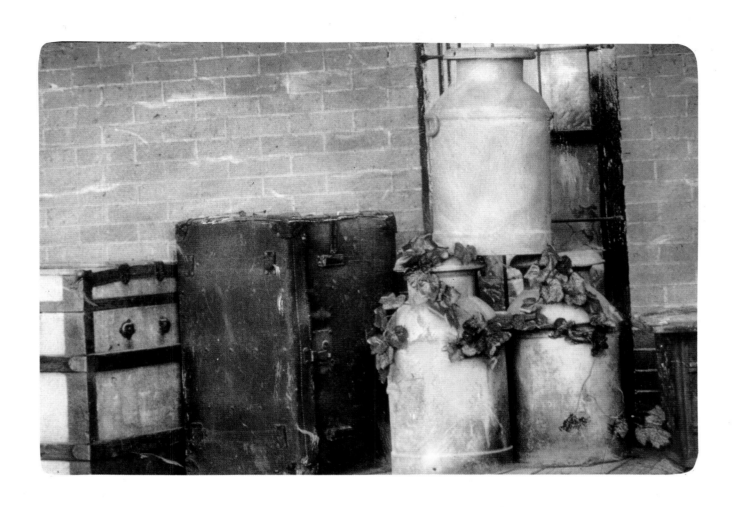

Untitled, 1990. Hand-painted C-print photograph, 12½ x 16 in.

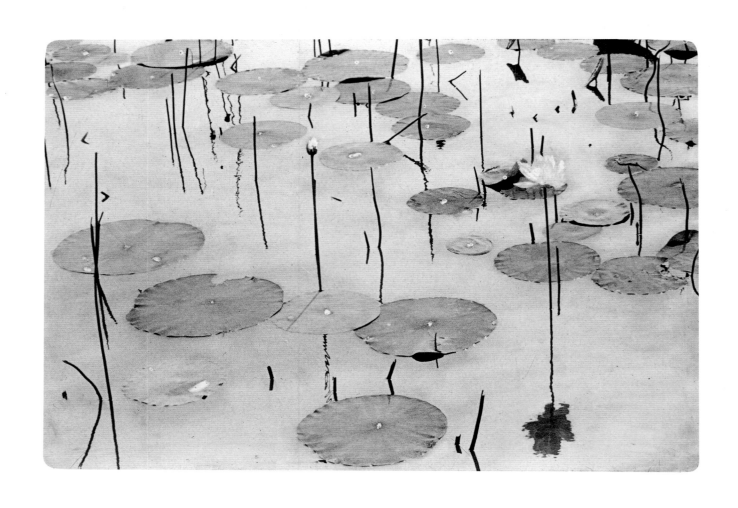

Untitled, 1991. Hand-painted C-print photograph, 19½ x 26 in.

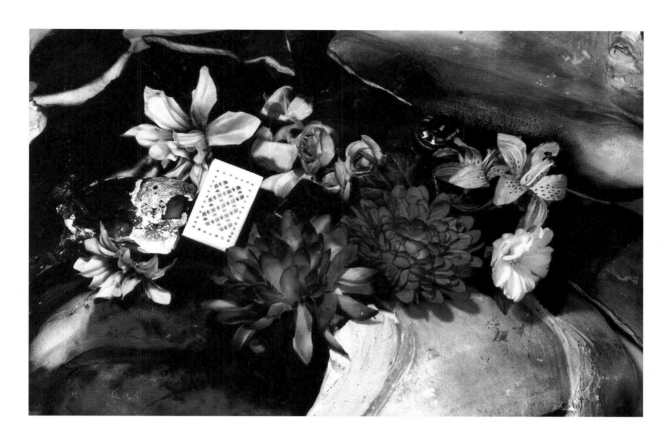

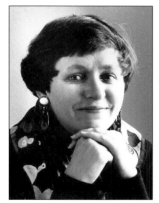

"Most people take focus for granted, but for me it is a vision that I have developed."

Kay Yasutome is a published poet who decided four years ago that she would learn photography to illustrate her manuscripts. "My ability to photograph and print," she explains, "comes directly from the demanding training that I pursued in my study of poetry with poet Sandra McPherson.... Be aware of the essential detail.... Create a tactile memory through both verbal and visual metaphor." Yasutome says she chooses to photograph still lifes because she likes to concentrate on what she can control "within the limits of my fifteen years of MS." Her work is frequently exhibited in Oregon.

Kay Yasutome

Portland, Oregon

Reassurance III, 1992. Black-and-white photograph, 16 x 20 in.

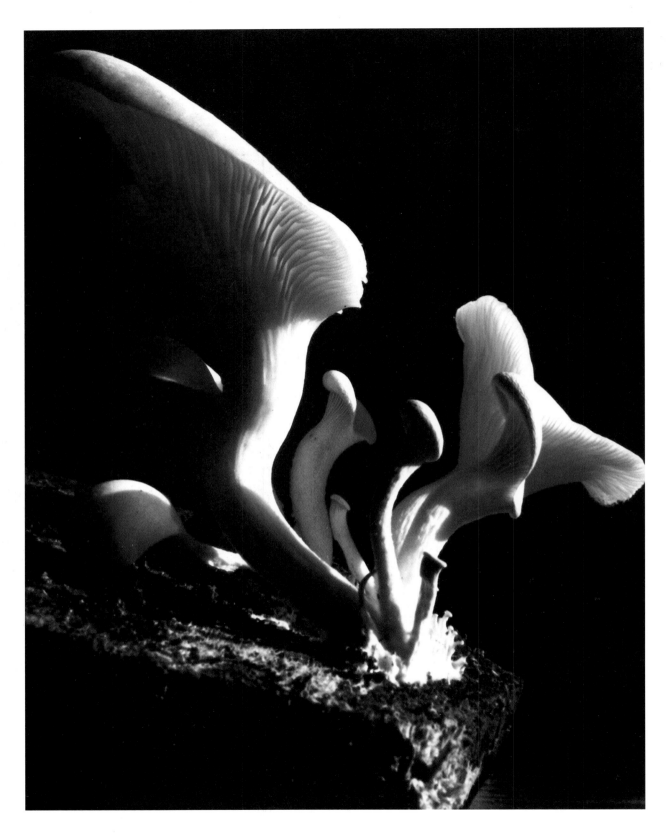

Diagonal, 1992. Black-and-white photograph, 20 x 16 in.

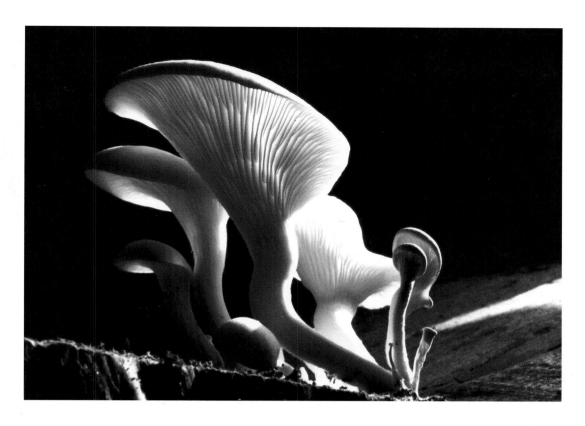

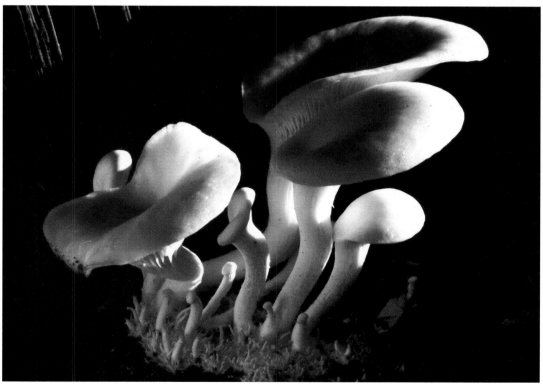

Radius, 1992. Black-and-white photograph, 16 x 20 in. (top) *Oval,* 1992. Black-and-white photograph, 16 x 20 in. (bottom)

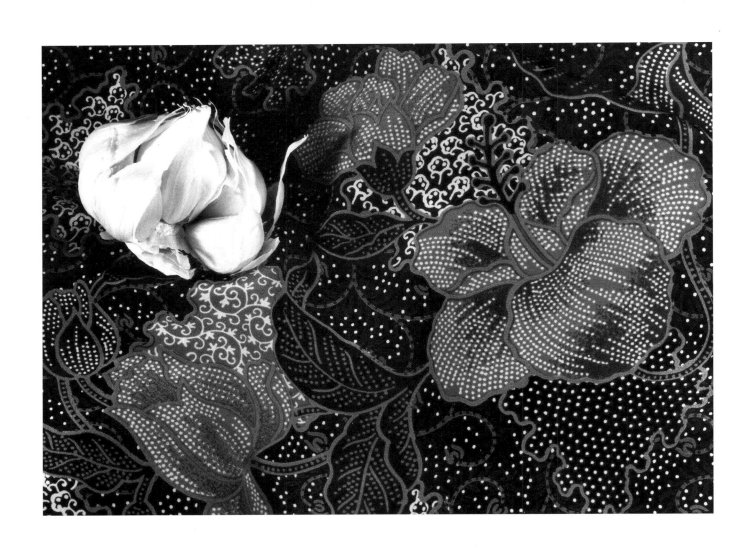

Garlic Moon, 1991. Black-and-white photograph, 16 x 20 in.

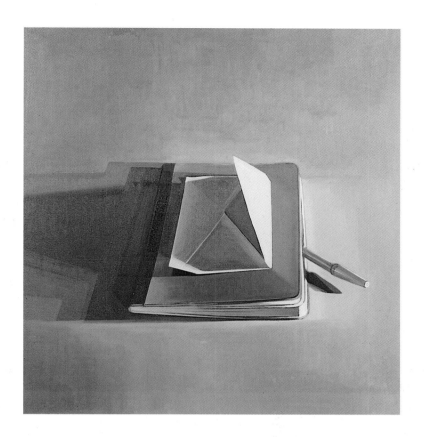

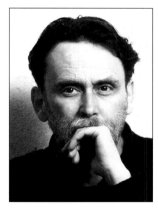

"These still-life paintings are about my belief in what I see and how I see. They are open-ended, ongoing emotional dialogues."

Hugh C. Yorty

Springfield, Missouri

Since 1966, when he was twenty-three, Hugh Yorty has exhibited his paintings. He describes himself as a painter of objects. "These paintings," he explains, "are not descriptions...but have content and psychological meaning.... They are as much about human drama as if there were figures in them." In 1991 Yorty was diagnosed with MS. Painting is now an even more important means through which he communicates, attempting to "achieve a sense of the unpredictable" in his work. He has been professor of art and design at Southwest Missouri State University in Springfield since 1967.

The Journal, 1991. Oil on canvas, 27½ x 25½ in. Collection of the artist.

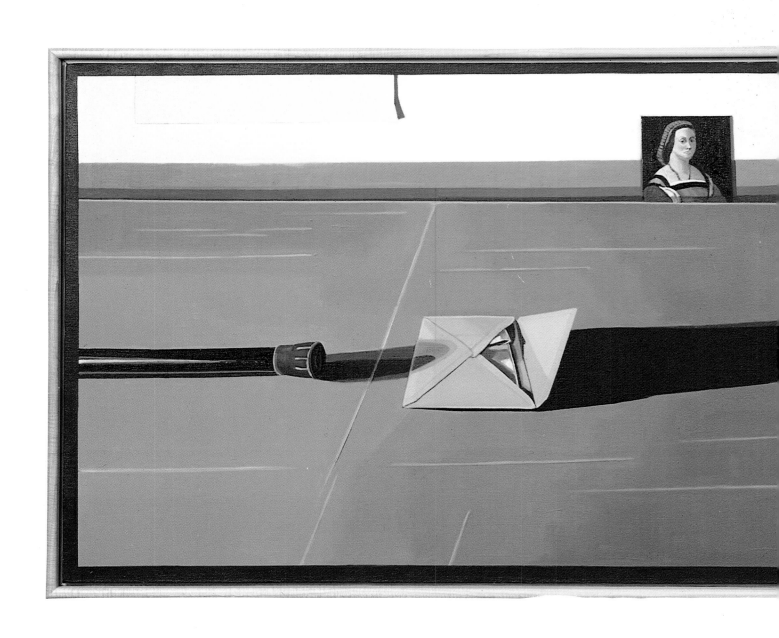

Two of My Canes and Two Letters Yet To Be Addressed, 1992. Oil on canvas, 25½ x 68½ in.

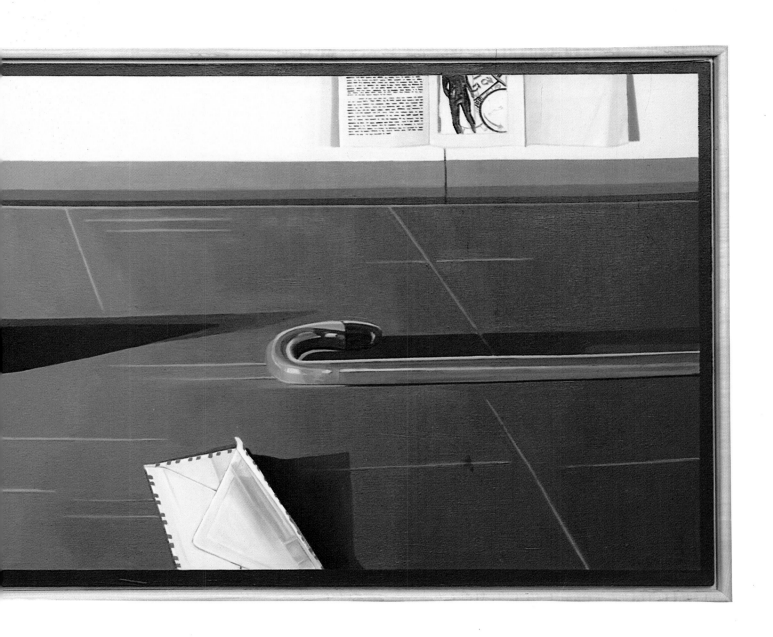

exhibition

Bess C. Bonner Colorado Springs, Colorado

Kalama, 1992. Oil on canvas, 20 x 16 in.
Spuzzum, 1992. Oil on canvas, 20 x 16 in.
Tahola, 1992. Oil on canvas, 16 x 20 in.
Unidentified Sea Creature, 1992. Oil on canvas, 20 x 16 in.

Karen L. De Witt Park Forest, Illinois

I feel so fine when they compare mine to Dine, 1992. Graphite, pastel and prisma on paper, 46 x 13½ in.
The Line Up, 1992. Graphite, pastel and prisma on paper, 21 x 46 in. Collection of Ann Benson
Mophead III, 1992. Graphite, pastel and prisma on paper, 46 x 36 in.

Laszlo Dus Brecksville, Ohio

Untitled, 1989. Handmade paper, 27 x 37 in.
Untitled (triptych), 1989. Acrylic on canvas, 36 x 69 in.

Victoria (Tori) Ellison Brooklyn, New York

Untitled, 1987. Acrylic on paper, 60 x 48 in.
Untitled, 1991. Wire, paint and steel shavings, 18 x 12 x 12 in.
Untitled, 1991. Wood, mirror, ash, wire, paint and plastic tubing, 5 x 13 x 13 in.

Leah Finch Margate, Florida

Cradle of Sustenance, 1992. Low fire ceramics, 16 x 18 x 4 in.
Untitled, 1992. Low fire ceramics, 12 x 23 x 18 in.

Phoebe Fuller-Graham Irvine, California

Origami Box #1, 1992. Watercolor on paper, 28¼ x 36 in.
Origami Box #2, 1992. Watercolor on paper, 28¼ x 36 in.
Summer Still Life on Batik #1, 1992. Watercolor on paper, 23¾ x 15¼ in.

Judith J. Hahn Woodinville, Washington

Ferns I, 1992. Watercolor on paper, 27 x 33 in.
Ferns II, 1992. Watercolor on paper, 33 x 37 in.

John M. Hall San Jose, California

Alex, 1991. Watercolor woodcut, 6 x 4½ in.
James At Home, 1991. Watercolor woodcut, 6 x 6 in.
Picasso Smiling, 1991. Watercolor woodcut, 5½ x 4 in.
Wild At Heart, 1991. Watercolor woodcut, 6 x 6 in.

Angelina M. A. Hekking
San Francisco, California

Another Relapse I Feel Devasted (Self-Portrait), 1984. Black-and-white photograph, 16 x 20 in.
Homeless People in Washington Square Park, S.F. (Self-Portrait), 1986. Black-and-white photograph, 16 x 20 in.
Homeless Person, "Homer" in Washington Square Park, S.F., 1986. Black-and-white photograph, 20 x 16 in.
Homeless Person, "Tim" in Washington Square Park, S.F., 1986. Black-and-white photograph, 20 x 16 in.

Thomas W. Hollender Nutrioso, Arizona

Cinder Pit #1, 1990. Mixed media on masonite, 96 x 120 in.
Untitled, 1992. Mixed media, 30 x 42 in.

Robert Otis Holter Scotts Valley, California

Kiss Me Quick in the Morning Mist, 1992. Acrylic on canvas, 48⅜ x 41⅛ in.
Portrait of a Victorian Lady, 1992. Acrylic on canvas, 61⅜ x 51 in.

Carol Hunt Southampton, New York

Remembered Suns, 1991. Oil on canvas, 66 x 90 in.
Improvisation (M4F2), 1992. Monotype, 36 x 24 in.
Improvisation (M4J2), 1992. Monotype, 53¼ x 38⅛ in.
Improvisation (M4J3), 1992. Monotype, 53¼ x 38⅛ in.
Zapote, 1992. Oil on canvas, 60 x 72 in.

James Iatridis Tenafly, New Jersey

Irene I, 1990. Acrylic on canvas, 20 x 16 in.
Travelers, 1990. Acrylic on canvas, 20 x 24 in.
Woman #1, 1991. Acrylic on canvas, 24 x 18 in.

Dina Kawer Huntington Woods, Michigan

Chinese Lacquer, 1992. Polaroid transfer image on Japanese kozo paper, 3¼ x 4¼ in.
Four Pears, 1992. Polaroid transfer image on Japanese kozo paper, 3¼ x 4¼ in.
Gladiolus, 1992. Polaroid transfer image on Japanese kozo paper, 3¼ x 4¼ in.
Roman Vessel, 1992. Polaroid transfer image on Japanese kozo paper, 3¼ x 4¼ in.
Tulips II, 1992. Polaroid transfer image on Japanese kozo paper, 3¼ x 4¼ in.

Frieda King   Long Beach, California

Reflections, 1990. Oil on canvas, 33 x 24 in.
Green Moon, 1992. Oil on canvas, 28 x 32¼ in.

Rona Ginn Klein   Abington, Pennsylvania

Self Portrait IV Revisited, 1992. Mixed media, 22 x 30 in.
Synergy I, 1992. Color laser print, 17 x 23 in.
Synergy II, 1992. Color laser print, 17 x 23 in.
Synergy III, 1992. Color laser print, 17 x 23 in.
Synergy IV, 1992. Color laser print, 17 x 23 in.

Jessie Jane Lewis   Philadelphia, Pennsylvania

Catskill Landscape, 1988. Oil on paper, 25½ x 33 in.
Electrical Circuits, 1989. Pastel and graphite on paper, 46½ x 34 in.
Pink Flesh Contacts, 1989. Pastel and graphite on paper, 44⅜ x 36½ in.

Linda L. Longo-Muth   Valley Cottage, New York

The Glass of '92, 1991. Acrylic on canvas, 49 x 41 in.
Made in the U.S.A., 1991. Acrylic on canvas, 49 x 41 in.
The Glass Ceiling, 1992. Acrylic on canvas, 41 x 49 in.
The Glass of '93, 1992. Acrylic on canvas, 49 x 41 in.
It's Your Choice, 1992. Acrylic on canvas, 49 x 37 in.
    Private collection.

Marty Manning   Fairfax, Virginia

Amaryllis Snow White, 1990. Watercolor and gouache on paper, 48 x 36 in.
Rose Bowl, 1990. Watercolor and gouache on paper, 22 x 30 in.

Thomas Martin   New York, New York

Employment, 1989. Oil on canvas, 24 x 36 in.
Ages 45 to 50, 1991. Oil on canvas, 60 x 48 in.

Ruby McLain   Fort Washington, Maryland

Fragile, 1989. Black-and-white photograph, 20 x 16 in.
Keep Quiet, 1989. Black-and-white photograph, 20 x 16 in.
Senses, 1990. Black-and-white photograph, 28 x 22 in.

Surel Mitchell   Boise, Idaho

AE-5, 1991. Acrylic on unstretched canvas, 60 x 57 in.
AE-6, 1991. Acrylic on unstretched canvas, 83 x 49 in.

Debra Norby   Portland, Oregon

Pond Water 2, 1992. House paint on wood, 48 x 48 in.
3 Women, 1992. House paint on wood, 24 x 24 in.
    Collection of Betsy Wolfston.
A Woman & A Man, 1992. House paint on wood, 24 x 24 in.

Mary O'Hara Gregory
   Philadelphia, Pennsylvania

A Classic, 1985. Color photograph, 20 x 24 in.
Just Put Your Foot Down, 1989. Color photograph, 20 x 24 in.

Jeana Sirabella   New York, New York

Carmela II, 1992. Oil on quilted fabric, 48 x 29 x 2 in.

Karen G. Stone   Albuquerque, New Mexico

Kivas, Coronado Ruins, 1988. Color photograph, 16 x 20 in.
Ranchos de Taos, 1988. Color photograph, 20 x 16 in.
Adobe Wall Detail, 1989. Color photograph, 16 x 20 in.

Charles Strouchler   New York, New York

Two Barns, 1989. Oil on paper, 23½ x 29 in.
Two Boats, 1989. Pastel on paper, 16½ x 18¾ in.
The Trees, 1990. Oil on paper, 22½ x 28¾ in.

James Uhl   Kingston, Pennsylvania

Dreaming, 1989. Color photograph, 12 x 15 in.
Hard Day's Night, 1989. Black-and-white photograph, 14 x 11 in.
Modesty, 1989. Color photograph, 12 x 15 in.
Nepalese Ragamuffins, 1989: Black-and-white photograph, 14 x 11 in.
Old Friends, 1989. Black-and-white photograph, 11 x 14 in.

Lorna R. Warden   Richmond, Virginia

Untitled, 1990. Hand-painted C-print photograph, 11 x 14 in.
Dancers, 1991. Hand-painted C-print photograph, 12½ x 16 in.
Untitled, 1991. Hand-painted C-print photograph, 19½ x 26 in.

Kay Yasutome   Portland, Oregon

Garlic Moon, 1991. Black-and-white photograph, 16 x 20 in.
Diagonal, 1992. Black-and-white photograph, 20 x 16 in.
Oval, 1992. Black-and-white photograph, 16 x 20 in.
Radius, 1992. Black-and-white photograph, 16 x 20 in.
Reassurance III, 1992. Black-and-white photograph, 16 x 20 in.

Hugh C. Yorty   Springfield, Missouri

The Journal, 1991. Oil on canvas, 27½ x 25½ in.
    Collection of the artist.
Two of My Canes and Two Letters Yet To Be Addressed, 1992. Oil on canvas, 25½ x 68½ in.

multiple sclerosis is a chronic disease of the central nervous system, which is typically diagnosed in young people between the ages of twenty and forty. Close to a third of a million Americans have MS, with women outnumbering men two to one.

All but a few people with MS can expect to live a normal life span, but many will do so with increasing levels of physical disability. Symptoms can range from slight blurring of vision to complete paralysis. The most common problems are fatigue, muscle weakness, problems with balance and gait, spasms, tingling numbness, and disturbances in bladder function.

The disease develops through immune system attacks on a fatty substance called myelin, which surrounds and protects nerve fibers. The resulting damage interferes with the passage of nerve impulses. The cause of MS is not yet known, but treatments are beginning to emerge from research; many symptoms can now be successfully managed, and hopes are high for definitive progress in the near future.

the national ms society, established in 1946, is the most comprehensive national resource for MS-related information in the United States. It is the only U.S. voluntary health agency supporting international research into the cure, cause, prevention and effective treatments for multiple sclerosis. Through a fifty-state network of 141 chapters and branches, the Society provides extensive program services to individuals with MS and their loved ones. Chapter services include education, counseling, advocacy, equipment assistance and information and referral.

For further information on multiple sclerosis and the Society you may call the 24-hour toll free information line, 1-800 LEARN MS, or write: National MS Society, 733 Third Avenue, New York, NY 10017.